Sterile Processing

FOR PHARMACY TECHNICIANS

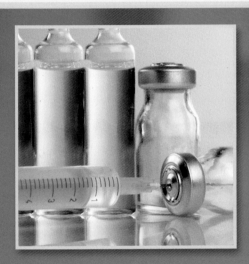
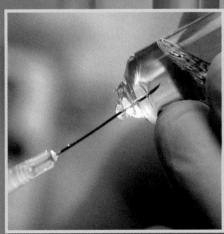

Karen Davis, AAHCA, CPhT

Chair of Pharmacy Technician and Surgical Technology Programs
Education Corporation of America
Virginia College
Birmingham, Alabama

ELSEVIER

SAUNDERS

3251 Riverport Lane
St. Louis, Missouri 63043

Vice President and Publisher: Andrew Allen
Executive Content Strategist: Jennifer Janson
Associate Content Development Specialist: Kate Gilliam
Associate Content Development Specialist: Elizabeth Bawden
Content Coordinator: Kevin Korinek
Publishing Services Manager: Julie Eddy
Project Manager: Jan Waters
Design Direction: Amy Buxton

Printed in China

Last digit is the print number: 9 8 7 6 5 4 3 2 1

Working together
to grow libraries in
developing countries

www.elsevier.com • www.bookaid.org

Reviewers

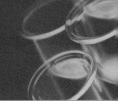

Julie E. Beccarelli, CPhT
Pharmacy Technician II
Chesapeake Regional Medical Center
Chesapeake, Virginia

Charles B. Fowler, RPh, BS Pharmacy
Lead Pharmacy Technician Instructor
Vantage Career Center
Van Wert, Ohio

Paula Lambert, CPhT, BS MEd
Pharmacy Technician Instructor
North Idaho College
Coeur d'Alene, Idaho

Joshua J. Neumiller, PharmD, CDE, CGP, FASCP
Assistant Professor
Department of Pharmacotherapy
College of Pharmacy
Washington State University
Spokane, Washington

Michelle D. Remmerden, RPT, CPhT, BS
Program Director—Pharmacy Technician
Everest University
Pompano Beach, Florida

WITHDRAWN

Preface

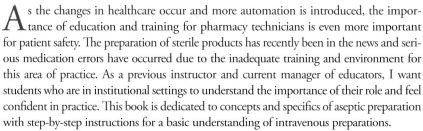

As the changes in healthcare occur and more automation is introduced, the importance of education and training for pharmacy technicians is even more important for patient safety. The preparation of sterile products has recently been in the news and serious medication errors have occurred due to the inadequate training and environment for this area of practice. As a previous instructor and current manager of educators, I want students who are in institutional settings to understand the importance of their role and feel confident in practice. This book is dedicated to concepts and specifics of aseptic preparation with step-by-step instructions for a basic understanding of intravenous preparations.

Preparers will use this book to learn the history and principles of aseptic technique, as well as learning the basic steps of sterile preparation. They will have guides for lab competencies and self-assessments to ensure a basic understanding before entering the field.

The more the pharmacy technicians understand aseptic practice, the safer all patients will be. It is imperative to maintain a sterile environment and provide a quality intravenous product. Technicians who go through this advanced practice will be validated and enter the pharmacy profession a step above other programs who just teach these concepts through lecture and demonstrations. The students will perform each major step in aseptic technique and will be able to perform at externship with minimal supervision.

ORGANIZATION

The book starts with the history of aseptic technique and then discusses the equipment, environment, and basic skills and techniques used. The progression allows the students to understand what and when they will use these skills, and then allows them to perform each step through a series of hands-on laboratory exercises, self-assessments, and critical thinking.

DISTINCTIVE FEATURES

The book is crosswalked to the ASHP goals and objectives and follows the most current version of the USP 797 guidelines. The students have detailed self-assessments as well as critical thinking and real world examples to ensure their understanding and performance of hands-on skills. These detailed checklists can be provided as documentation for ASHP accredited programs as well as prospective employers.

LEARNING AIDS

A variety of pedagogical features are included in the book to aid in learning:
- **Learning Objectives** listed at the beginning of each chapter clearly outline what students are expected to learn from the chapter materials.
- A list of **Key Terms** follows the Learning Objectives and identifies new terminology and makes it easier for students to learn this new vocabulary; learning this new terminology is vital to success on the job.

- **Tech Alerts** are found in the margins of the text and alert the student to drug look-alike and sound-alike issues.
- Helpful **Tech Notes** are dispersed throughout the chapters and provide critical, need-to-know information regarding dispensing concerns and interesting points about pharmacology.
- **Lab Activities** allow students to perform basic aseptic manipulations in lab.
- **Competency Checklists** provide measurable outcomes that reflect master of the task.
- **Review and Critical Thinking Questions** further enhance student review and retention of chapter content by testing them on the key content within the chapter.
- The **Reference List** provides a list of sources that students and instructors can use for additional information on the chapter's topic.

ANCILLARIES

FOR THE INSTRUCTOR
Evolve

We offer several assets on the Evolve website to aid instructors:

- **Test Bank:** An ExamView test bank of multiple-choice questions that feature rationales, cognitive levels, and page number references to the text. This can be used as review in class or for test development.
- **PowerPoint Presentations:** One PowerPoint presentation per chapter. These can be used "as is" or as a template to prepare lectures.
- **Image Collection:** All of the images from the book are available as JPGs and can be downloaded into PowerPoint presentations. These can be used during lectures to illustrate important concepts.
- **Text Answer Key:** All of the answers to the Review and Critical Thinking questions from the text are available.
- **TEACH:** This includes lesson plans and PowerPoint slides, all available via Evolve. TEACH provides instructors with customizable lesson plans and PowerPoints based on learning objectives. With these valuable resources, instructors will save valuable preparation time and create a learning environment that fully engages students in classroom preparation. The lesson plans are keyed chapter-by-chapter and are divided into logical lessons to aid in classroom planning. In addition to the lesson plans, instructors will have unique lecture outlines in PowerPoint with talking points, thought-provoking questions, and unique ideas for lectures.

Note to Students

The pharmacy technician is such an incredible and important part of healthcare and the pharmacy industry. Never stop learning and progressing in your career. This book will allow you to complete a program with an advanced understanding of intravenous preparation, and employers will seek that out. The sky is the limit and I am living proof. You may want to write and teach one day, and there is no reason you can't. I encourage you to gain as much knowledge as you can, and institutional practice is a great field to work towards.

Acknowledgment and Dedications

I would like to dedicate this book to the first Pharmacist, Billy Kittrell, who taught me intravenous preparation almost 20 years ago. I have had many great mentors along the way in my career, and to each of them, I would also like to say "thank you." I would also like to say thank you to the Elsevier team who have been more supportive than I could ever imagine. Also, a special thank you to my family, especially my husband, who has always encouraged me and tells me every day that he is proud of me. I couldn't have done this without each of you.

Karen Davis, AAHCA, CPhT
Birmingham, Alabama

Contents

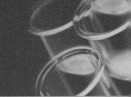

1

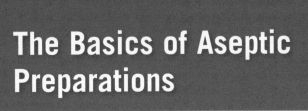
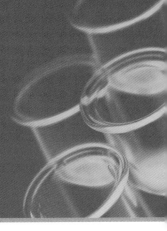

The Basics of Aseptic Preparations

LEARNING OBJECTIVES

1. Explain why certain medications must be sterile.
2. Discuss the history of aseptic preparation and the organizations that provide guidelines.
3. Define the term *aseptic technique,* and demonstrate proper handwashing procedures.
4. Discuss the responsibilities, regulations, and workplace settings of personnel who compound parenteral preparations.

TERMS & DEFINITIONS

Asepsis Condition free from germs, infection, or any form of life

Centers for Disease Control (CDC) United States Federal Agency under the Department of Health and Human Services concerned with control and prevention of diseases

Compounded sterile preparations (CSP) Medications prepared using sterile technique

The Joint Commission The shortened term for the Joint Commission on Accreditation of Healthcare Organizations; a nonprofit, private organization that evaluates medical facilities to ensure good patient care

Normal flora Bacteria that resides on the skin's outer surface but does not cause disease

Microorganism An organism (such as a bacterium, virus, or protozoan) of microscopic size

Parenteral Any medication route other than the alimentary canal (digestion system)

Pyrogen Fever producing substance

Standard precautions CDC guidelines that promote hand hygiene and the use of personal protective equipment (PPE)

Sterile Free of living organisms, especially microorganisms

United States Pharmacopoeia (USP) Nongovernmental, not for profit public health organization that set standards for over-the-counter (OTC) and prescription medicines and other health care products in the United States; its main goal is to ensure public health

USP 797 Chapter in the USP concerning parenteral medications compounding and equipment endorsed by The Joint Commission and American Society of Health-System Pharmacists (ASHP)

INTRODUCTION

Pharmacy technicians must have a good understanding of aseptic technique and the practices surrounding the preparation of sterile products to ensure safety, accuracy, and correctness of the medication. In this chapter we will discuss the history and concept of asepsis, along with the regulations and responsibilities of personnel who prepare intravenous admixtures (Figure 1-1). We will also discuss handwashing and the correct performance procedure according to the **Centers for Disease Control (CDC)** guidelines. Following the proper procedures is the only way to ensure that contamination does not occur when performing aseptic technique.

The art of compounding aseptic or **sterile** preparations has been performed since the beginning of pharmacy. Pharmacy personnel must prepare intravenous medications when other routes, such as oral tablets or liquids, may not be appropriate because the patient cannot take them by mouth or in emergency situations where rapid absorption is required. This route is known as **parenteral,** which is derived from two Greek words; *para* meaning around and *enteron* meaning the intestines. These medications must be free from **pyrogens** or microbes that cause infection since they are administered directly into the body via the blood and bypass many of the body's natural defenses.

Patients receiving intravenous medications are often hospitalized and immune compromised, and they are more susceptible to infection (Figure 1-2). Since sterile intravenous products can be prepared in many settings, such as hospitals, outpatient pharmacies and clinics, doctor's offices, and in a patient's home, the need for extremely clean or sterile preparation is imperative to ensure the wellbeing of these patients. Typically, the normal bacteria that we all have on the surfaces of our body do not affect us because we are healthy, but to a sick person these can cause significant harm, and since patients receiving intravenous therapy are usually the most critical, every precaution must be taken to avoid contamination. The personnel responsible for their preparation must follow certain rules and guidelines as well as use specialized

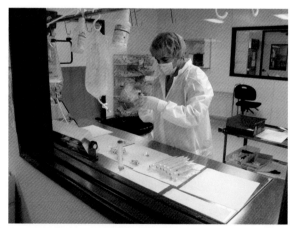

FIGURE 1-1 A technician in a hospital intravenous room. (From Hopper T: *Mosby's pharmacy technician: principles & practice,* ed 3, St Louis, 2012, Saunders Elsevier.)

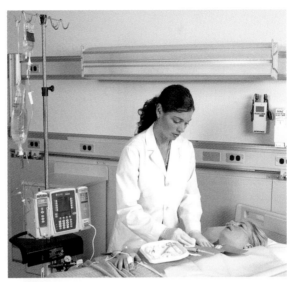

FIGURE 1-2 A patient receiving intravenous therapy in a hospital. (Courtesy of CareFusion, San Diego, CA.)

equipment. Technicians perform most of the preparation duties today under the direct supervision of a pharmacist.

History of Aseptic Preparations

The practices of medicine advanced very quickly during the early nineteenth century and researchers discovered that germs and unknown organisms caused certain diseases. In the 1600's people believed that ***microorganisms*** spontaneously came from decaying nonliving matter.

Louis Pasteur's germ theory in the early 1800's specified that bacteria caused diseases (Figure 1-3). Practices that are common today, such as handwashing, were not practiced routinely. As a result, many deaths were attributed to the unclean conditions of operating rooms and personnel practices. A person was more likely to die of postoperative gangrene than the surgery itself. As a result, many changes in the practices were established. In 1865, Sir Joseph Lister, a well-known surgeon, read a paper by Louis Pasteur and learned about the germ theory of disease. He stated that if infections were caused by microbes, the best way to prevent infections would be to kill the microbes before they reached the open wound. Lister used carbolic acid to kill germs. He wrote about the use of this acid in his work, *Antiseptic Principle of the Surgery Practice.* (essortment.com)

The use of sanitary dressings and instruments led to the development of disposable supplies, such as syringes, needles, and other intravenous supplies in the 1920's (Figure 1-4). Sterile solutions and equipment became accepted in health care in the 1930's. In the 1960's, following a rash of serious patient complications, the National Coordinating Committee on Large Volume Parenterals (NCCLVP) published the first set of recommendations for pharmacy and other health care professionals. In 1972, the Baxter Corporation produced a training manual which was later revised in 1990.

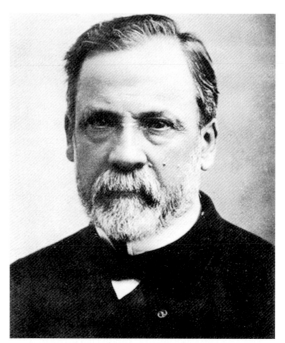

FIGURE 1-3 Louis Pasteur, 1822-1895. (From US National Library of Medicine, Bethesda, MD)

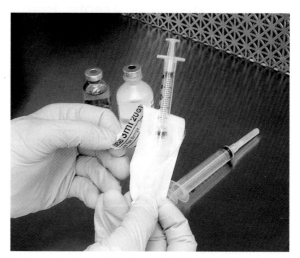

FIGURE 1-4 Packaged syringe. (Courtesy of CriticalPoint, LLC, Gaithersburg, MD)

Following these guidelines, American Society of Health-System Pharmacists (ASHP) and *United States Pharmacopoeia (USP)* published updated guidelines that are considered standard practices for pharmacy personnel when preparing sterile preparations or *compounded sterile preparations (CSPs).*

Aseptic technique is required when preparing any medication that enters the body through a parenteral or ophthalmic route. According to the *USP 797,* these preparations may include compounded biologics, diagnostics, drugs, nutrients, radiopharmaceuticals, eye preparations, and tissue implants.

Bacteria are stained with a substance called *crystal violet.* Those that retain the color are gram positive, and those that lose the color are gram negative. Antibiotic drugs are grouped together or classified based on their activity against gram positive organisms, such as staphylococci (Figure 1-5), or against gram negative organisms, such as aminoglycosides activity against diplococci (Figure 1-6). Once the bacteria is determined to be gram positive or gram negative, a physician can prescribe the medication that works most effectively for either a gram positive or a gram negative bacteria.

Today, industry standards for the preparation of intravenous products include the use of proper practices or aseptic technique, specific procedures, equipment, training of personnel, and storage recommendations. These guidelines are provided by the USP, which is an official standards-setting organization made up of a volunteer body of experts in the medical field. Chapter 797, which was written in 2004, was the first enforceable document to outline the practices associated with sterile compounding. These guidelines were recently updated and continue to provide the best practices associated with sterile preparation of intravenous medications. In the 1980's, the document known as *ASHP Guidelines on Quality Assurance for Pharmacy-Prepared Sterile Products by the American Society of Health-System Pharmacists* was published and supported the USP 797 guidelines for the pharmacy industry. Both of these organizations address quality assurance activities for CSPs and are endorsed by **The Joint Commission** on Accreditation of Hospitals. The Joint Commission is a nonprofit organization that accredits more than 16,000 health care organizations and programs in the United States. Their main focus is on patient rights, treatment, and infection control. The purpose of the USP 797 and ASHP guidelines is to describe practices and environmental conditions that prevent harm or even death to patients.

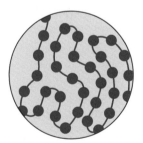

FIGURE 1-5 Gram-positive bacteria.

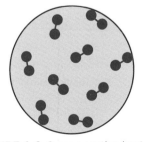

FIGURE 1-6 Gram-negative bacteria.

To achieve these standards, the guidelines provide minimum practices and quality standards and include:

- Policy and procedures for compounding
- Provision of records or documentation as part of an ongoing quality assurance program
- Proper training of pharmacists and technicians in aseptic technique
- Provision of reference materials
- Separate facilities and air quality controls to ensure that sterile conditions are available for aseptic compounding
- Establishment of storage and beyond use dates for sterile products
- Hygiene procedures to include garb and handwashing

Aseptic Technique

Aseptic technique refers to manipulation of medications or fluids from one container to another, and its primary goal is to maintain *asepsis* or keep all products free from contamination from microbes. This requires special training, special procedures, and special equipment. The personnel preparing aseptic products must always remember to keep any potential harm from coming to the patient.

According to the CDC, the first line of defense against the spread of microorganisms is good handwashing. There are always bacteria present on our bodies and hands known as *normal flora.* These bacteria are a basic defense mechanism for our bodies and are found on the skin, in the vagina, and intestines. Some, such as *E. coli,* are necessary in the digestive process in the colon. However, to a patient who has an immune compromised system, they can cause harm, infection, and even death, because the person is susceptible to infection as a result of their alteration in normal immune function.

HANDWASHING AND STANDARD PRECAUTIONS

One of the most important aspects of proper aseptic technique is proper handwashing. The most common type of contamination is touch, and since we have bacteria on our body surfaces at all times, it is important to avoid the transfer of these to any product going directly into a person's bloodstream. Organizations, such as the CDC, have standards known as *standard precautions* for the health care industry to prevent the transfer of microorganisms. This organization is a government agency that is part of the Department of Health and Human Services. Their main task is to formulate safety guidelines concerning the spread of infection, which is a significant part of aseptic technique guidelines.

Here are some key points to remember for handwashing:

- Always wash your hands before entering the clean room or after doing anything that may contaminate the hood, such as eating or performing personal hygiene tasks.
- Remove all jewelry, and use a suitable antibacterial agent to scrub hands up to elbows. See the CDC guidelines for approved products.
- Turn on water, and wet hands and forearms thoroughly while holding them upward.
- Be sure to wash in between fingers and under nail beds.
- Thoroughly rinse and dry hands, and then turn water off with a lint free paper towel (Figure 1-7).

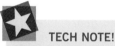

TECH NOTE!
Staphylococci is a naturally occurring bacteria or type of normal flora present on our hands all the time.

TECH NOTE!
The route of administration for parenteral medications is directly into the bloodstream; therefore, injectable medications must be prepared aseptically always remembering the increased risk of infection.

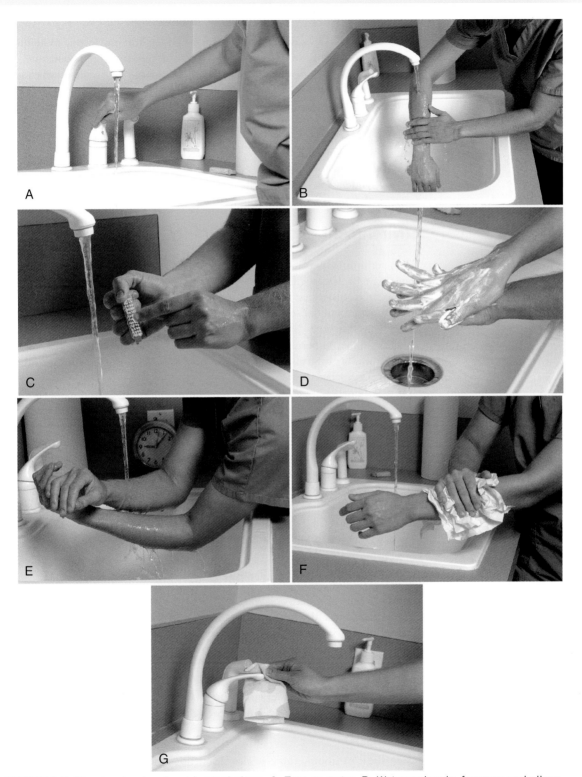

FIGURE 1-7 Step-by-step handwashing technique. **A.** Turn on water, **B.** Wet your hands, forearms and elbow, **C.** Clean underneath your fingernails, **D.** Soap your hands, **E.** Rinse your hands thoroughly, **F.** Dry your hands, **G.** Turn off water. (From Salvo SG: *Massage therapy: principles and practice,* ed 3, St. Louis, 2007, Saunders)

The observance of handwashing precautions and performing aseptic technique is imperative to ensure patient safety and the sterility of the intravenous admixture. The result of a compromised admixture can result in a nosocomial infection, which is an infection the patient receives during health care treatment. This can eventually lead to death and significant costs to the health care system.

PERSONAL PROTECTIVE EQUIPMENT

Along with proper handwashing and aseptic technique, wearing appropriate personal protective equipment (PPE) is also required. Personnel compounding or performing aseptic technique must wear sterile gloves, gown, protective eyewear, mask, beard covers, and shoe covers. We will discuss the procedures for their use in Chapter 8.

Environment and Responsibility of Personnel

When performing aseptic technique, there are basic duties that intravenous or compounding technicians will be responsible for. These are determined by the facility's policies and procedures as well as industry standards. This will usually include preparation techniques, calculations, data entry and labeling, and delivery. Even though the pharmacist must provide the end check, that does not mean that the technician is not responsible for being as accurate and correct in the procedure as they can possibly be. This takes a conscientious and detailed approach to technique and proper preparation.

It is extremely important that the finished product is free of contaminates and correctly prepared and labeled. As part of the USP 797 guidelines, there should be a quality control (QC) or quality assurance (QA) program in place to include validation of performance, preparations, and environmental controls. This should be a written evaluation to assess the compounding personnel's performance when preparing aseptic preparations as well as cleaning procedures and validation of equipment and devices. Once this is in place, it will provide a mechanism to monitor, evaluate, and improve the activities and processes used. The first step in any QC program is knowledge. Knowing about the medications and using strict aseptic technique throughout the entire process will ensure a safe product for the patient.

CLEANROOM AND AIR SPACE

Another important aspect of aseptic manipulations is the environment in which it must be performed. The controlled area is normally referred to as a *class 100 environment* according to standards set by the ASHP and USP 797. These standards refer to a cleanroom in which the air temperature, quality, and humidity are highly regulated in order to prevent cross contamination. The air is continuously filtered and is a positive pressure room. This means the outside air that is unfiltered and dirty is not allowed inside the cleanroom. The designated area or room should be away from the flow of regular traffic and only authorized, trained personnel should be allowed.

THE HOOD

Inside the cleanroom, there is also an airflow hood called a *laminar airflow workbench (LAFW)* where aseptic manipulations take place. This horizontal

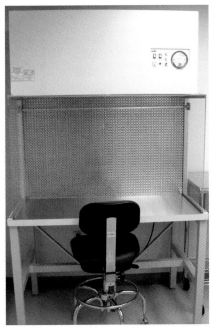

FIGURE 1-8 A laminar airflow workstation (LAFW). (Courtesy of CriticalPoint, LLC, Gaithersburg, MD)

flow hood provides a clean space with constant air filtration through a special filter called a *high-efficiency particulate air (HEPA) filter* (Figure 1-8). The room air is drawn into the hood through a pre-filter and then through the HEPA filter at the back of the hood. This filter removes particles that are 0.2 microns or larger, which is nearly all bacteria and fungi that is present. This filtered air is then blown horizontally or across the work surface toward the front of the hood.

Biological safety cabinets (BSCs) that have vertical airflow are also used when compounding hazardous drugs and will be discussed in Chapter 6 (Figure 1-9).

Settings for Intravenous Therapy

The administration and preparation of sterile products most often occurs in an institutional setting, such as the hospital, but can also take place in a long-term care facility, retail pharmacy, and even physicians' offices. Since the population of older people is increasing due to the extended life expectancy, there is often a need for home health intravenous therapy, and these medications are prepared in a facility and delivered to the patient's home. It is imperative that the preparer have a good understanding of the medications, their storage, techniques when preparing, and delivery systems being used, such as pumps. Patient education should also be stressed, especially in a home health care setting.

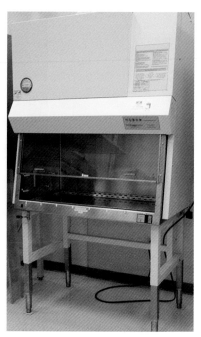

FIGURE 1-9 Biological safety cabinets (BSCs). (Courtesy of CriticalPoint, LLC, Gaithersburg, MD)

REVIEW
QUESTIONS

1. Discuss why parenteral medications must be prepared using aseptic technique.
2. List at least three considerations covered by USP 797 concerning the preparation of CSPs, and explain why they are important.
3. According to USP 797, name three types of CSPs that require aseptic |preparation.
4. List at least three elements of a quality assurance (QA) program, and discuss why they are important.
5. List three duties that a compounding or intravenous technician will be responsible for.

CRITICAL
THINKING

1. You are a technician supervisor at a large hospital and recently have hired two new technicians for the intravenous room. How would you explain why using aseptic technique is imperative to the hospital patient's health?
2. Using the following website, list at least four groups of people who are most likely to acquire a gram negative infection, and explain why. http://www.upmc.com/patients-visitors/education/infection-control/Pages/gram-negative-infection.aspx

3. You are a technician supervisor for the local hospital. Recently, a technician student asks you, "Why are most of the supplies used when preparing intravenous drugs disposable? Doesn't that cost a lot of money?" How would you explain the cost effectiveness of disposable supplies over reusable supplies like syringes and needles?

COMPETENCIES
THE BASICS OF ASEPTIC PREPARATIONS

Evaluation Key: S= Satisfactory   NI= Needs Improvement

Name: Quarter: Date:

COMPETENCIES	STUDENT			INSTRUCTOR		
Student will be able to:	**S**	**NI**	**Comments**	**S**	**NI**	**Comments**
Define aseptic technique.						
Discuss USP 797 guidelines and the importance of these standards.						
List preparations included in USP 797 that are considered compounded sterile preparations (CSPs).						
Discuss the basis for using parenteral medications.						
Discuss the importance of normal bacteria and why it does not cause infection in healthy persons.						
Discuss handwashing technique and its importance.						
Discuss the responsibilities of a compounding technician.						
Discuss settings where parenteral medications may be administered.						
Discuss elements of a quality assurance (QA) program and its importance.						

Review each concept to ensure that the learning objectives for the chapter have been met. Your instructor or supervisor will evaluate this as well.

LAB ACTIVITY

Evaluation Key: S= Satisfactory   NI= Needs Improvement

Name: Quarter: Date:

COMPETENCIES	STUDENT			INSTRUCTOR		
Student will be able to:	S	NI	Comments	S	NI	Comments
Remove all jewelry, (i.e., rings, watches, and bracelets).						
Adjust water to lukewarm (not hot).						
Wet hands under running water.						
Apply antimicrobial liquid soap, and rub hands together.						
Work soap into lather by adding water, and rub for 2 minutes.						
Cover all surfaces of hands, including sides, backs, and palms.						
Interlace the fingers, and move soapy water between them.						
Keep hand pointed upward, keeping hands and forearms at or below elbow level.						
Rinse hands thoroughly under running water taking care to not touch sink or faucets.						
Dry each hand with a clean paper towel, and discard towels.						
Turn the faucet off with a *new dry* towel and discard.						

Bibliography

1. Pharmaceutical compounding-sterile preparations (general information chapter 797). In: The United States Pharmacopeia, 27th rev. and The National Formulary, 22nd ed. Rockville, MD: The United States Pharmacopeial Convention, 2004:2350-70.
2. American Society of Health-System Pharmacists: ASHP Guidelines on Quality Assurance for Pharmacy-Prepared Sterile Products. Accessed March 1, 2013 at http://www.ashp.org/s_ashp/docs/files/BP07/Prep_Gdl_QualAssurSterile.pdf
3. Centers for Disease Control and Prevention: Guideline for hand hygiene in health-care settings: recommendations of the healthcare infection control practices advisory committee and the HICPAC/SHEA/APIC/IDSA hand hygiene task force, *MMWR* 51(RR-16:2, 29-33). October 2002: http://www.cdc.gov/mmwr/PDF/rr/rr5116.pdf. Accessed March 1, 2013.
4. *Dorland's illustrated medical dictionary*, ed 31, Philadelphia, 2007, Saunders.
5. Sir Joseph Lister: Developer of Antiseptic Surgery. *essortment* (website): http://www.essortment.com/sir-joseph-lister-developer-antiseptic-surgery-37935.html. Accessed March 1, 2013.
6. Mitchell J, Haroun L: *Introduction to health care*, ed 2, Clifton Park, NY, 2007, Thomson Delmar Learning.
7. The Joint Commission: *Facts about the Joint Commission* (website): http://www.jointcommission.org/about_us/fact_sheets.aspx. Accessed March 1, 2013.
8. usp797.org, inc.: *Welcome to USP797.org* (website): http://www.usp797.org/index.html. Accessed March 1, 2013.
9. The United States Pharmacopeial Convention: *USP & Healthcare Professionals* (website): http://www.usp.org/audiences/healthcarePro/healthcareProviders.html. Accessed March 1, 2013.

2

Administration of Intravenous Products

1. Identify the types of parenteral medications and nutrition, and name at least three situations where it would be beneficial to use a parenteral dose form.
2. Describe two types of intravenous (IV) administration, and give an example of each.
3. Name two advantages and two disadvantages of administering IV medications.
4. Discuss the types of parenteral medications and supplies used in both health-system IV administration and home infusion therapy, and explain the technician's integral role in preventing medication errors when considering administration of parenteral medications.

TERMS & DEFINITIONS

Bolus Also known as *direct injection* or *intravenous push (IV push; IVP)*; small amount of medication injected into a port usually in an existing IV line

Epidural injection Injection into the epidural space

Intra-arterial injection Injection into an artery

Intracardiac (IC) injection Injection into the cardiac muscle or the heart

Intradermal (ID) route Injection into the dermal layer of the skin

Intramuscular (IM) injection Injection into the muscle

Intrathecal (IT) route Injection into the spinal canal

Intravenous (IV) injection Injection into the vein

IV push (IVP) Also known as *bolus*; small amount of medication injected into a port usually in an existing IV line

Lactated Ringer's solution (LR) Sterile isotonic intravenous fluid used for electrolyte or fluid replacement

Normal saline (NS) Sterile intravenous solution, also known as sodium chloride, used as a source of water or for fluid replacement

Subcutaneous route of administration (Sub-Q) Injection just below the skin into the subcutaneous fat layer

INTRODUCTION

Pharmacy technicians must have a good understanding of routes of administrations for parenteral medications. Certain drugs are available in limited forms and require special considerations when mixing with fluids and performing aseptic technique. In some cases there are even medications that can only be administered one way and require special equipment that must be included with the prepared admixture. In this chapter we will discuss patient considerations, some advantages and disadvantages of parenteral therapy, and types of infusions in an effort to avoid potential errors that may occur if not considered.

Parenteral Medications and Nutrition

Medications that are given intravenously bypass the digestive processes. These medications reach the bloodstream almost immediately and can be useful in emergency situations where fluid replacement is needed and another dosage form is not appropriate. A parenteral dosage form may be administered several ways, including methods such as intravenous (IV), intramuscular (IM), intracardiac (IC), and intrathecal (IT).

Intravenous (IV) injection medications are administered directly into the bloodstream through a vein. It is the most common parenteral route, and it has rapid effects. Injections can be via a syringe and needle, or in some cases through a pump or programmable machine, such as for pain or diabetes control. This route is administered either through a peripheral line or a central line. A peripheral line goes into the extremities, such as the arm, hands, and feet.

Peripheral veins are smaller, which allows medication to be injected easier. This is the most common method of administration. A central line is used for a weak patient or one who has weak peripheral veins. Medications, such as total parenteral nutrition (TPN) or chemotherapy, are usually too concentrated for peripheral veins and are given centrally through an implanted port because there is more blood volume running through these larger veins.

Intramuscular (IM) injections, such as hormones, vaccinations, and some antibiotics, are given directly into the muscle. *Intracardiac (IC) injection* medications are usually used in emergencies and typically found on emergency or crash carts. These medications, such as epinephrine, are often used quickly to resuscitate a patient and therefore are packaged in prefilled disposable syringes with attached needles. The *intradermal (ID) route* is used to inject medications in the capillary rich layer below the epidermis, such as in a skin test for tuberculosis. The *intrathecal (IT) route* is used for injections directly into the space surrounding the spinal cord. Meningitis patients often receive injections through the IT route when a spinal tap is performed. All medications given through this route are preservative free because the body may not be able to break them down, which could cause permanent paralysis. *Intra-arterial injections* may be used to inject anesthesia medications or dyes into an artery during a procedure, such as a heart catheterization. The *subcutaneous route of administration* is used for slowly absorbed medications like insulin or heparin.

TECH ALERT!
The abbreviation SQ or SC should not be used for subcutaneous because it could be mistaken for SL or sublingual and increase the chance of an error. You can find a list of "DO NOT USE ABBREVIATIONS" on The Joint Commission website at *http://www.jointcommission.org/assets/1/18/Do_Not_Use_List.pdf.*

A direct injection, often called a *bolus* or *IV push (IVP),* is a small amount of medication in a syringe injected directly into a port in an existing IV line over 5 to 15 minutes, such as a pain medication. Pain or nausea medications for a hospital patient may be injected through the IV line for patients who already have an IV line inserted. This type of injection allows the patient to receive necessary medications without the additional "stick" or puncture.

Epidural *injections* are given into the epidural space, such as anesthesia medication during labor.

Oral dosage forms must pass through the digestive processes to reach the bloodstream and be distributed to the organs and tissues.

Some drugs, such as heparin (an anticoagulant), are broken down completely by stomach acids and for this reason must be given parenterally. Therefore, much of what determines the best route of administration is due to the drug's effectiveness. There are also diseases or conditions that lead to the inability of a patient to be able to take an oral dose form, such as a tablet or an oral solution. These may include patients who are:

- Unconscious
- Experiencing extreme nausea and vomiting
- Unable to swallow a tablet, such as a child or elderly patient
- Uncooperative due to illness, such as psychiatric disorders
- Experiencing a life-threatening situation, such as blood loss, where immediate replacement intervention is required
- Unable to absorb medication through the gastrointestinal (GI) tract due to disease
- Extremely dehydrated

Intravenous Administration

There are different types of IV administration. An IV injection can be a small amount of medication in a syringe injected directly into the vein through the skin, such as a pain medication. This method is called *IV push.* Sometimes these are injected directly into a port in an existing IV line to avoid an additional puncture in the skin. If a larger amount of medication is need, it may be given as an IV infusion. This is designed to allow the medication to flow into the bloodstream over a longer period of time, such as in a blood transfusion or antibiotic treatment, which takes about 30 minutes.

IV medications may be given continuously or intermittently. This is usually in the form of a large volume parenteral (LVP) between 250 to 1000 mL and over 2 to 24 hours. The orders will determine a rate of infusion, which is the amount of fluid that should enter the body over a certain period of time (Figure 2-1). This is often regulated with an infusion pump or electronic device. Examples of IV injections include hydration fluids, blood products, or drugs that need to be maintained at a constant or steady level for the patient.

Intermittent infusions are volumes of fluid from 25 to 250 mL and are often infused from 15 to 90 minutes at specific intervals. These drugs can be given in between a continuous infusion and often through the existing tubing if there are no compatibility

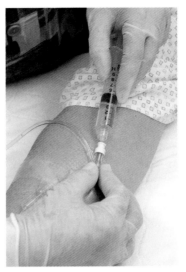

FIGURE 2-1 Infusion; larger amount of medication needed, such as with a blood transfusion or administration of antibiotics. (From Ogden SJ, Fluharty LK: *Calculation of drug dosages: a work text,* ed 9, St Louis, 2012, Elsevier Mosby.)

issues with the drugs themselves. Examples include an antibiotic ordered at 6 hours over 30 minutes. This drug would be mixed in a small amount of fluid, such as dextrose or sodium chloride, and administered at specific intervals.

IV push (IVP) is another method of administration (Figure 2-2). This is often referred to as *direct administration* and is used to administer high concentrations of medications, such as those needed for pain. This route is prepared aseptically and packaged in a syringe for administration. The dose is injected directly into the skin, but often can be given through an existing port in the person's IV tubing. This is a

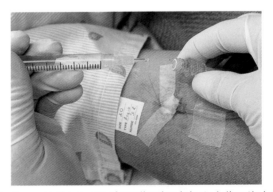

FIGURE 2-2 Push; a small amount of medication injected directly into a vein, such as with pain medication. (From Ogden SJ, Fluharty LK: *Calculation of drug dosages: a work text,* ed 9, St Louis, 2012, Elsevier Mosby.)

way to prevent another needle puncture for the patient and decrease the risk of infection and additional pain.

ADVANTAGES OF INTRAVENOUS MEDICATIONS

All medications must reach the blood and be distributed before they can be beneficial. Since parenteral doses of medication do not have to be processed through the digestive system, they are able to reach their intended organ or tissue rapidly. This is the greatest advantage, and for this reason IV injection is often used in emergency situations. Even antibiotics are given this way if there is a necessity to prevent the spread of infection quickly.

Other advantages of IV injections include:

- Drugs, such as insulin and heparin, that normally would be destroyed in the stomach can be administered.
- There is a rapid onset of action, which means the medications take effect and begin to work fast (for example, relieving a high fever in a child).
- Patients receiving treatment therapy, such as dialysis, surgery, chemotherapy, or epidurals, can receive medications parenterally.

DISADVANTAGES OF INTRAVENOUS MEDICATIONS

Since drugs pass through a normal body's protective barrier and go directly into the bloodstream, there can be many complications. There is a significant risk of infection due to the entrance of a needle into the skin. This opening to the outside of the body allows a place for microbes to enter and cause an infection. Common adverse reactions to IV therapy include phlebitis and infiltration. *Phlebitis* is an inflammation of the vein and can cause symptoms such as burning, redness, pain, and stinging. Infiltration can also occur, which is when the fluid goes into the tissue surrounding the vein at the injection site. Both of these conditions must be considered when administering IV medications.

There is always the "fear of being stuck by a needle" to consider and pain that accompanies IV medication therapy.

The effects of an error in parenteral medications are also a disadvantage. If an error or an interaction with the drug occurs, it is impossible to remove the medication immediately from the body because it is in the bloodstream. This often means the patient will have to wait for the effects to wear off.

The cost of IV therapy is also a consideration. As discussed previously, these medications must be prepared aseptically by trained personnel and often require administration by home health nurses or hospitalization.

Health-System Intravenous Administration

IV therapy can be given in the hospital, in long-term care facilities (such as nursing homes), during emergency transport, in hospice, and in doctor's offices.

Medications can include hydration infusion, antibiotic therapy, nutritional therapy, pain management, and chemotherapy. Often a pump or electronic device is used to administer these fluids in order to regulate the infusion safely and accurately. Pumps used for pain therapy or diabetes management can be portable or even implantable (Figure 2-3).

TECH NOTE!
Since heparin is available in 10 units/mL, 100 units/mL, 1000 units/mL, and 10,000 units/mL and is considered a "high alert" drug, it is extremely important to double check all dosages through either a second person or other protocol established by your facility.

TECH NOTE!
The opening in the skin created by the puncture needle presents significant risk for an infection, such as phlebitis.

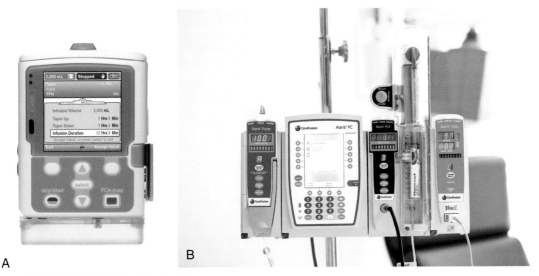

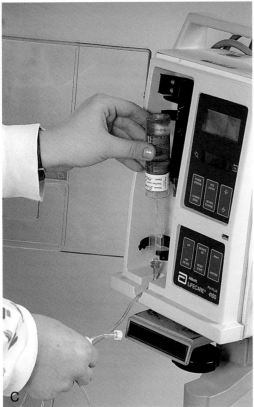

FIGURE 2-3 Electronic infusion devices. **A,** CADD-Prizim VIP ambulatory battery-operated infusion device used for IV parenteral nutrition. **B,** Medley™ Medication Safety System. **C,** Nurse using a patient-controlled analgesia (PCA) electronic infusion device. (**A,** Courtesy of Smiths Medical ASD, Inc., St Paul, MN. **B,** Courtesy of CareFusion, San Diego, CA. **C,** From Potter PA, Perry AG: *Fundamentals of nursing,* ed 6, St Louis, 2005, Mosby.)

Home Infusion Therapy

The supplies, including the pump, for IV therapy are delivered along with the IV medication. Generally, technicians are responsible for maintaining these devices and supplies.

Some of the supplies needed include:
- IV start kits (Figure 2-4)
- IV tubing
- Syringes and needles
- Alcohol swabs
- Sharps container
- Gloves
- Batteries

All of these supplies are provided as part of the infusion delivery, and patients or family members can often administer these with nursing support. In long-term care or hospice, the nurse or a trained caregiver administers these IV medications once they are prepared by a technician or pharmacist using aseptic technique. It is imperative that a technician include all the supplies, such as pumps or tubing, needed to administer the medication so that the nurse or caregiver has what they need. Without the proper additional supplies (such as tubing, syringes, needles, and solutions used to flush the IV tubing), the nurse cannot administer the medication properly, and the patient will be unable to receive treatment.

The pharmacy technician or preparer must consider the route of administration to be used and the setting where it will be given when preparing parenteral

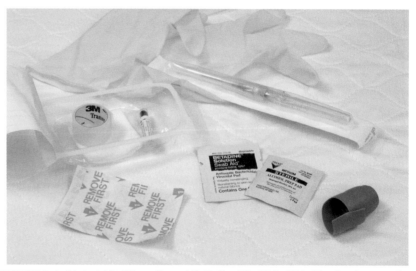

FIGURE 2-4 IV start kit. (From Perry AG, Potter PA, Elkin MK: *Nursing interventions & clinical skills,* ed 5, St Louis, 2012, Elsevier Mosby.)

medications. Whether the medication is to be given continuously, intermittently, or via IVP requires certain packaging and preparation methods. The health care team, starting with the preparer and ending with the patient, must consider IV therapy complications, such as phlebitis. Infection control begins with good aseptic technique and is the first step in quality management. Familiarity of the drugs, their preparation, and routes of administration are all factors in preventing medication errors and ensuring the patient is safe.

REVIEW QUESTIONS

1. Name two advantages of IV administration.
2. Name two disadvantages of IV administration.
3. Name two different types of IV therapy that might be given in the home infusion pharmacy.
4. Name three types of patients who would need to receive IV therapy.
5. Which parenteral route results in the fastest onset of drug action because it goes directly into the bloodstream?
6. Name a drug which must be given parenterally due to destruction by stomach acids if taken orally.

CRITICAL THINKING

For the following orders, determine what type of infusion they are considered to be and why:
1. The order reads:
   Give ampicillin 500 mg in NS 100 mL over 15 minutes every 6 hours.
2. The order reads:
   Give dextrose 1000 mL IV every 12 hours for 3 days.
3. The order reads:
   Give 25 mg promethazine (Phenergan) IV for nausea and vomiting stat.
4. The order reads:
   Give LR 1000 mL ✕1 for dehydration.

COMPETENCIES
ADMINISTRATION OF INTRAVENOUS MEDICATIONS

Evaluation Key: S= Satisfactory   NI= Needs Improvement

Name: _____   Quarter: _____   Date: _____

COMPETENCIES	STUDENT			INSTRUCTOR		
Student will be able to:	**S**	**NI**	**Comments**	**S**	**NI**	**Comments**
Discuss parenteral routes of administration.						
Discuss types of settings where IV medication would be appropriate.						
Discuss the advantages and rationale for using IV method of administration over oral forms.						
Discuss types of patients or conditions that parenteral routes are indicated for use in.						
Describe infiltration and phlebitis and why they occur.						
Interpret a physician's order to distinguish which entries are IV drugs.						
Using provided reference materials, determine the route of administration that would be appropriate for the medication ordered.						
Explain why it is important for the preparer to know the route of administration of an IV when preparing it for a patient.						

LAB ACTIVITY

Order 1

512333 OB-1 05/26/05 Davis, Karen Dr. Davis 05/28/13 Obstetric	Diet _____WT_____HT_____ Diagnosis _____gestational diabetes_____ Drug Allergies __NKA_____
05/28/13 0600	Admit pt, consult Debbie for diabetic teaching Ampicillin 1 gm IV q8h 1st dose now LR c 20 mg KCL at 125 mL/hr Toradol 30 mg IVP q6h Repeat CBC and potassium level in AM Vitals q4h while awake 1800 cal diet V/o Dr. Davis/ Mrs. Jones

CBC, Complete blood count; *IVP*, IV push; *KCL*, potassium chloride; *LR*, lactated Ringer's solution; *NKA*, no known allergies; *pt*, patient; *V/o*, vocal order.

Order 2

512333 OB-1	Diet _____WT____HT____
05/26/05	
Davis, Karen	Diagnosis <u>Pre-op</u>_____
Dr. Davis	
05/04/13	Drug Allergies ____NKA_____
PACU	
05/05/13 0700	Admit pt to PACU
	Give Narcan 0.4 mg immediately
	Toradol 30 mg IVP on arrival to PACU and repeat q6h for a total of 3 doses prn pain
	Ancef 1gm IV q6h
	Phenergan 25 mg IV or IM q6h prn for itching
	LR @125 mL/hr
	Vitals q4 while awake
	V/o Dr. Davis/ Mrs. Jones

IM, Intramuscular; *IV*, intravenous; *IVP*, IV push; *LR*, lactated Ringer's solution; *NKA*, no known allergies; *PACU*, post-anesthesia care unit; *prn*, as needed; *pt*, patient; *V/o*, vocal order.

Using the physician's orders above, answer the following questions:
1. List the IV medications prescribed.
2. Which IV medication is a continuous infusion?
3. Which IV medication is an antibiotic? What type of infusion is this?
4. Are there any medications that could be given as IV push? If so, which ones, and what are they for?

Bibliography

1. Pharmaceutical compounding-sterile preparations (general information chapter 797). In: The United States Pharmacopeia, 27th rev. and The National Formulary, 22nd ed. Rockville, MD: The United States Pharmacopeial Convention, 2004:2350-70.
2. Wallace L. *Basics of aseptic compounding technique video training program*, ed 1, Bethesda, MD, 2006, American Society of Health-System Pharmacists.
3. Davis K, Sparks J. *Getting started in non-sterile compounding video training program*, ed 1. Bethesda, MD, 2007, American Society of Health-System Pharmacists.
4. The Joint Commission: *Facts about the Official "Do Not Use" List* (website): http://www.jointcommission.org/assets/1/18/Do_Not_Use_List.pdf. Accessed March 1, 2013.

3

Medications Used in Intravenous Preparations

1. Discuss the four processes of pharmacokinetics that parenteral medications go through.

2. Discuss factors that must be considered when determining the correct dosages for parenteral medications, including why pediatric and elderly patients require special dosing considerations.

3. Name at least two references to use to find the storage requirements for a parenteral medication.

TERMS & DEFINITIONS

Absorption Movement of a drug into the circulatory system

Adverse effects Drug effects that are unexpected and unwanted and are usually reported in only a few patients

Distribution Movement of a drug through the body into tissues, membranes, and then organs

Excretion Removal of a drug from the body

Metabolism Changing of the chemical structure of a drug by the body

Side effects Drug effects that are predictable, widely reported, and can be found in literature

Therapeutic effect The intended effect of a drug

INTRODUCTION

Technicians are required to prepare intravenous (IV) admixtures using aseptic technique with the correct fluids and knowledge of what they are for and how they react in the body. Medications often have special considerations because of the processes they go through in the body. A technician must be aware of the medication's properties, its interactions and side effects, and any special considerations that need to be followed when preparing the drug to ensure patient safety and medication accuracy. In this chapter, we will discuss concepts of pharmacokinetics, dosing information, and the references that are available.

Pharmacokinetics for Parenteral Medications

Manufacturers create medications with the ability to release and be distributed over a certain period of time. The process that drugs go through in the body is known as *pharmacokinetics* and includes four different steps. The first step is known as ***absorption.*** This process is the movement of the drug through barriers, such as the digestive tract, into the bloodstream where it can be distributed to the target organs or tissues. With parenteral medications, there are no barriers to slow the movement of drugs into the bloodstream because they bypass these digestive processes. This allows the second step or ***distribution*** of drugs to occur. This distribution process is what allows the drug to reach its target cells and exert its action. Target cells have special places where drugs go to allow a specific action to take place. These places are known as *receptor sites.* This is sometimes referred to as a "lock and key" mechanism, which describes the interactions of the drug at the receptor sites on the target cell (Figure 3-1).

Everything happens at a cellular level, and since parenteral forms of medications are injected into the bloodstream and are allowed to bypass natural defenses, such as the gastrointestinal tract, they reach the target cell quickly. Drugs have to reach the blood and be distributed before they act on the body. The third step in the drug's life is to be metabolized in the liver, and this is an actual chemical alteration of the original drug. The primary enzyme system responsible for ***metabolism*** is the cytochrome P450. ***Excretion*** is the fourth and last phase of a drug's life, and often occurs in the kidneys. Drugs are eliminated from the body a number of ways but most commonly through urine, feces, breast milk, and sometimes sweat.

If a drug is given intravenously, it bypasses the gastrointestinal (GI) system and goes directly to the bloodstream where it is distributed throughout the body. When a drug is given via an intramuscular (IM) injection, it is absorbed through tissue membranes and then enters the bloodstream (Figure 3-2).

Drugs administered orally must be absorbed in the stomach before reaching the blood for circulation. This is why IV medications have the most rapid onset of action or begin to work the fastest.

Special Dosing Considerations for Parenteral Medications

The dose of a drug is the amount of drug given at one time, and this varies with each patient. The recommended dose of a drug to produce the desired effect is known as

Check Out Receipt

UA Lane Road
614-459-0273

Wednesday, January 11, 2023
1:09:44 PM
94946

Item: 31963003195569
Title: Sterile processing for
pharmacy technicians / Karen
Davis
Due: 2/1/2023

Total items: 1

You saved $110.00 by using
your library today.

For personalized service from
information experts...Start Here!
www.ualibrary.org

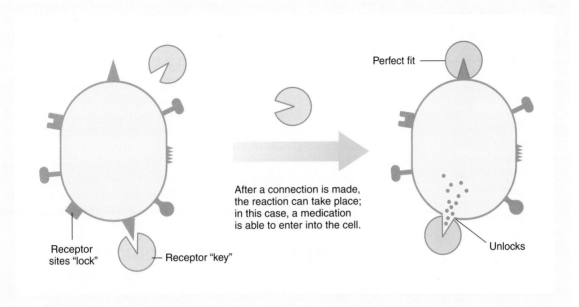

After a connection is made, the reaction can take place; in this case, a medication is able to enter into the cell.

Perfect fit

Unlocks

Receptor sites "lock"

Receptor "key"

FIGURE 3-1 The "lock and key" mechanism of receptor sites. (From Hopper T: *Mosby's pharmacy technician: principles & practice,* ed 3, St Louis, 2012, Elsevier Saunders.)

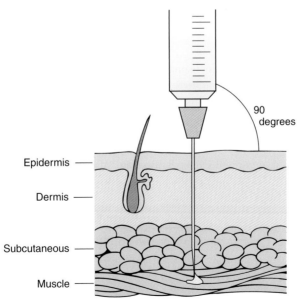

90 degrees

Epidermis

Dermis

Subcutaneous

Muscle

FIGURE 3-2 An intramuscular (IM) injection. (From Clayton BD, Stock YN, Cooper SE: *Basic pharmacology for nurses,* ed 15, St Louis, 2010, Mosby Elsevier.)

TECH NOTE!

When drugs are given to a patient, all three types of effects may occur. Adverse drug reactions (ADRs) should be reported to the US Food and Drug Administration (FDA) through their system known as *MedWatch* (http://www.fda.gov/medwatch/). A special FDA program to report ADRs for vaccines is called the *Vaccine Adverse Event Reporting System (VAERS)*.

the *therapeutic effect.* This means the dose given will be the most effective. If too little of a dose is administered, it can be subtherapeutic, which means it is not enough to be effective. If too much of a dose is administered, it can cause toxic or adverse effects, or in extreme cases be fatal.

All drugs produce certain effects, wanted and unwanted, including therapeutic effects, side effects, and adverse effects. Therapeutic effects are the desired effects of the drug. The dose required to achieve the desired therapeutic effect is somewhere between the smallest effective dose that can be given and the largest dose that is safe. *Side effects* can be found in the manufacturer's literature for a medication and are usually widely reported. Side effects are what patients experience from using the medication or during clinical trials. Common side effects include nausea, dizziness, and dry mouth. *Adverse effects* are usually unexpected and often require a dose change or possibly stopping the drug altogether. These effects may cause harm to the patient and with parenteral medications are even more dangerous because these drugs enter the bloodstream directly.

DISEASE STATES OR EXISTING CONDITIONS

Certain types of patients are considered contraindicated and should not take certain forms of medications. When dosing a patient, individual factors must be taken into consideration.

A patient may have other diseases that may affect the processes of pharmacokinetics, such as liver, kidney, or cardiovascular disease. If the liver does not function properly due to impairment caused by a disease or a decrease in function due to deteriorating body functions (the aging process), drugs may not be metabolized properly. If there are cardiovascular problems, the blood supply may be less than normal for the distribution process. If the kidneys have failed, drugs will not be excreted or removed from the body at the correct rate. This could mean a smaller dose would be required due to the impairment of vital organs.

AGE

Low weight in neonates and infants usually causes a reduction in the dosage of medication, but there are many other factors to consider when dosing medication for these patients (Box 3-1).

Neonates and infants have smaller skeletal structures, and this can affect the absorption of medication just as much (Figure 3-3). Since there is limited physical activity in these patients, there is a decrease in blood flow to the muscles. This causes slower absorption of the medication and increases the risk of muscle and nerve damage with

BOX 3-1   **Age Variables**

> Neonates—up to one month after birth
> Infant—between one month and 2 years
> Child—between age 2 and 12 years
> Adolescent—between 13 and 19 years
> Adult—between 20 and 70 years
> Elderly—older than 70 years

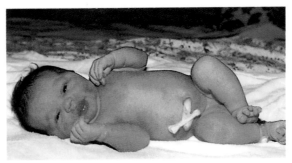

FIGURE 3-3 A neonate. (From Thibodeau GA, Patton KT: *The human body in health & disease,* ed 5, St Louis, 2010, Mosby Elsevier.)

any IM injection, since the medication is not absorbed into the bloodstream as quickly as with an adult. Several factors, such as blood flow and metabolism, influence how much of a drug reaches its organ or area of the body. Various organs, such as the liver and kidneys, have the largest blood supply.

In addition, the adult brain has a protective barrier called the *blood brain barrier,* which protects it from water-soluble substances. Drugs must have a certain degree of lipid- or fat-solubility to penetrate this barrier and get to the brain. Liver function and the blood brain barrier are still immature in pediatric patients, and they have a higher percentage of body water and a lower percentage of body fat than adults. If a lipid-soluble drug is administered to a pediatric patient, there is decreased distribution of the drug to the organs and body tissues due to the lower percentage of fat in the body. This causes more of the medication to stay in the blood longer, causing higher drug blood levels. In comparison, a water-soluble drug can cause lower drug blood levels when administered because the percentage of water is higher in the body, and there is more peripheral drug, distribution as a result.

Plasma protein in pediatric patients is lower than in adults, and this allows more of a drug to remain unbound or "free" in the body. Since only unbound medications exert a drug effect, the pediatric patient may have a greater intensity of a drug effect. The liver and the kidneys are not fully developed in pediatric patients. This causes metabolism and excretion to occur more slowly than in adults and allows the drug to stay in their body longer. Since the drug stays in the child's body longer, this can lead to a build-up of the drug, causing toxicity.

Elderly patients experience many differences in the pharmacokinetic processes as aging occurs (Figure 3-4). Cardiac output decreases significantly with age, which affects the amount of blood that the kidneys and liver receive. Since these organs should have the most blood flow, along with the brain, the metabolism and excretion processes are slower in this population, which allows the drug to stay in the body longer potentially leading to drug accumulation and toxicity. Drug distribution is greatly affected in the aging adult because the percentage of lean body mass or muscle and the total percentage of body water are lower than in the younger adult. Drug concentration levels in the body are less because there is less water for a drug to be distributed in. Since the amount of body fat increases with age, lipid- (fat-) soluble drugs are widely distributed in those organs that contain the most adipose

TECH ALERT!
According to the FDA, benzyl alcohol, a preservative in bacteriostatic water for injection, which is used regularly to dilute some powder forms of IV medication, has been associated with toxicity in neonates.

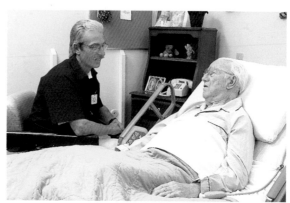

FIGURE 3-4 A geriatric patient. (From Sorrentino SA: *Mosby textbook for nursing assistants,* ed 6, p. 92, Fig. 6-8, St. Louis, 2004, Mosby.)

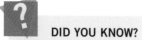

DID YOU KNOW?
Foods like broccoli act as a natural blood thinner and patients taking anticoagulants, such as warfarin (Coumadin), must avoid large amounts of these foods and other leafy green vegetables.

TECH ALERT!
Medications, such as heparin and insulin, are considered high alert drugs due to the dosing and the significant chance of causing harm to a patient. For a list of the most common high alert medications, see the Institute for Safe Medication Practices website, http://www.ismp.org/Tools/highalertmedications.pdf.

tissue. This causes the drug to be diverted from the kidneys and liver where the metabolism and excretion processes should take place. This slows the elimination of the drug from the body and causes it to have a longer half-life and toxicity due to the increased levels of medication in the bloodstream. Elderly patients are generally more sensitive to medications than younger people. This sensitivity often requires a reduction in the usual adult dosage. In an elderly person, the same dosage amount may produce a greater pharmacological effect.

DRUG INTERACTIONS

Drug-drug and drug-food interactions are also a concern. Often drug interactions will occur, and this can be a significant problem with parenteral medications. Since the medication enters the bloodstream and distribution occurs almost immediately, the effects can be magnified. Once the medications are administered, stopping their effects is almost impossible. Some drugs will potentiate the effects of another. In other words, the drug prolongs or magnifies the effect of another being given at the same time. An example would be a sleep aid that acts on the central nervous system combined with drinking alcohol. Some drugs, when given together, can increase each other's effects, such as naproxyn and aspirin, and may require a decreased dosage of both drugs to get the desired therapeutic effects. There are some drugs that negate the action of another, which is known as *antagonism*. These drugs may not be taken together, such as azithromycin (Zithromax) and antacids like Rolaids and Maalox.

There are also drug-food interactions. This occurs when a food affects the effectiveness or safety of a drug. Heparin is an IV anticoagulant and should not be taken with broccoli because they both thin the blood, and together they may cause internal bleeding.

BODY WEIGHT

The amount of drug required is related to weight because it determines the concentration of drug in the body. Pediatric patients, for instance, do not weigh what an average adult weighs, and dosages need to be adjusted. Formulas using body weight are often used to calculate a pediatric dose.

ROUTES OF ADMINISTRATION

There are some drugs that cannot be given orally due to the breakdown that occurs in the GI system. For example, heparin is destroyed by stomach acid and therefore is only available in injectable form.

Injectable medications have to be in an aqueous solution form to allow them to be injected into the body. They may be packaged as a solution and require preparation using a syringe to withdraw the desired amount; or, they may be packaged as a powder, which requires dilution with a specific fluid called a *diluent*.

The injectable medications will either be transferred to an IV solution container of fluid, usually in a plastic bag, drawn up in a syringe for IV push, or be manufactured as a ready-to-use premixed product. Examples of products available today are prefilled syringes, vials, or heat-sealed glass containers known as *ampules*. All of these products are considered sterile, and all manipulations require aseptic technique (Figure 3-5).

References and Storage Information

All drug products have a National Drug Code (NDC) for identification (Figure 3-6). This enables the technician to verify the exact product, because it identifies the specific drug, the manufacturer, and the package size.

The packaging information is the best source of information regarding the medications. The label of every drug package must include the following information:
- Brand and generic name
- Liquid forms of medications include the total volume of the container and the concentration, such as 25 mg/mL

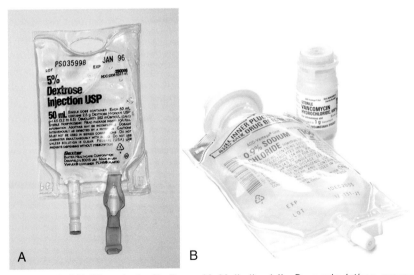

A   B

FIGURE 3-5 A-B, IV products. (**A,** Brown M, Mulholland JL: *Drug calculations: process and problems for clinical practice,* St. Louis, 2007, Mosby Elsevier. **B,** Courtesy Hospira Inc., Lake Forest, IL.)

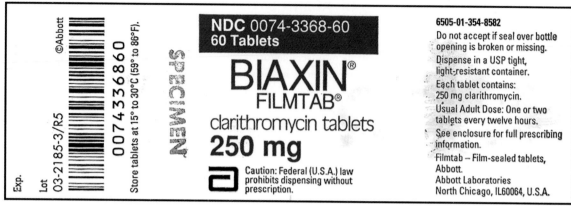

FIGURE 3-6 The National Drug Code (NDC) appears on this vial. (From Ogden SJ, Fluharty L: *Calculation of drug dosages: a work text,* ed 9, St Louis, 2012, Elsevier Mosby)

- Powder forms provide the information required to dilute the powder, including the concentration and directions for reconstituting the drug
- If it is a prescription medication, the label reads "Federal Law Prohibits Dispensing Without a Prescription" or "RX ONLY"
- Name and address of manufacturer
- Precautions associated with the drug
- Possible side effects and adverse effects
- Storage requirements, including refrigeration information, if needed

Other common reference sources to use for IV medications include *Drug Facts and Comparisons 2014,* the *Physicians' Desk Reference,* and the *Handbook on Injectable Drugs* by Lawrence A. Trissell. *Drug Facts and Comparisons* and the *Handbook on Injectable Drugs* contain the most current drug information. The *Handbook for Injectable Drugs* is used mostly in the hospital setting because it provides comprehensive compatibility information in chart form, such as what fluids a medication can be added to, storage requirements, stability, and preparation directions. In addition to these references, there are some quick-reference compatibility charts that some hospitals or facilities may use based on the literature made available from the manufacturers.

Technicians must be familiar with the content for various references in order to verify information about medications. These references are provided at the facility and should be updated continuously to ensure the most recent information. There are also continuing education lessons offered in magazines, such as "Drug Topics," "Pharmacy Times," and other publications, that are designed for technicians to stay current with the latest marketed drugs.

TECH ALERT!
Always be sure to check the source of printed charts or quick references by examining the medication package insert and/or consulting with a pharmacist. Remember to use a source you recognize and verify.

REVIEW
QUESTIONS

1. Name the four processes of pharmacokinetics.
2. Name two reasons why pediatric patients must be dosed differently from adults.
3. Name two reasons why elderly patients must be dosed differently from adults.
4. List two reference sources for parenteral medications and what type of information might be found in each.

CRITICAL
THINKING

1. Your patient is a 67-year-old woman who weighs 97 pounds. She has been diagnosed in the past with kidney problems. She presents to the emergency room complaining of extreme nausea and vomiting. She is dehydrated and needs fluids immediately. Your choice for medication is promethazine (Phenergan) IV or PO. Which route would you use, and why? Would the average adult dosage be appropriate? Why or why not?
2. Your patient is a 6-year-old child weighing 45 pounds. She presents to the emergency room with a rash, and the mother states that she had received a phenobarbital injection for seizures approximately 2 weeks ago but has recently started being irritable and unable to sleep through the night. Just last night, they noticed her slurring her words and became concerned. What type of effects do these reactions indicate? What should be done, if anything, for this patient?
3. The use of digoxin, a heart medication, has been associated with an increase in risk of falls in the elderly patient as well as an increase of toxic effects. Explain why this may occur. (Use a drug reference for your drug information.)
4. Using a drug reference of your choice, answer the following questions:
   • What is the generic name for Synagis?
   • What is it used to treat?
   • Explain how it is packaged and prepared for injection.
   • Name one contraindication for using Synagis.
   • Can this medication be used in pediatric patients?
   • How should this medication be stored?

COMPETENCIES

PATIENT CONSIDERATIONS FOR
INTRAVENOUS MEDICATIONS

Evaluation Key: S= Satisfactory   NI= Needs Improvement

Name: Quarter: Date:

COMPETENCIES	STUDENT			INSTRUCTOR		
Student will be able to:	**S**	**NI**	**Comments**	**S**	**NI**	**Comments**
Discuss the processes of pharmacokinetics for parenteral medications.						
Discuss the differences in pediatric patients and the need for dose adjustment.						
Discuss the differences in elderly patients and the need for dose adjustment.						
Discuss factors that must be considered when using IV medications.						
Identify at least two reference sources for IV medication information.						
Discuss side effects, adverse effects, and therapeutic effects and the differences.						
Using provided reference materials, identify drug information, such as storage, indications, contraindications, how supplied, NDC number, and interactions.						

LAB ACTIVITY

1. Using the online resource, GLOBALRPh, at www.globalrph.com, search for "New Drug Approvals," and list the brand and generic names of two drugs under the cardiology category. Then, discuss the mechanism of action, therapeutic use, usual adult dosage, and classification.

2. Using the online resource www.pdr.net (*Physicians' Desk Reference*), answer the following questions about Chantix: What is the generic name? What is the indication? What is the therapeutic class? Is this drug available in an injectable form? Name an adverse effect. Name a drug interaction.

3. Did you know that the American Association of Retired Persons (AARP) has a pill identifier option available online? Go to http://healthtools.aarp.org/pill-identifier, and enter the following information found on a medication brought in by a patient, under the imprint and shape section: **44 175** for the imprint and **capsule** for the shape. What drug is listed here? What classification of drug is it?

Bibliography

1. *Drug facts and comparisons* 2013, ed 68, Philadelphia, 2013, Lippincott Williams & Wilkins.
2. *Physicians' desk reference*, 2013 edition, Montvale, NJ, 2012, PDR Network.
3. *Taber's cylopedic medical dictionary*, ed 22, Philadelphia, 2013, F.A. Davis Company.
4. Trissel LA. *Handbook on injectable drugs*, ed 15, Bethesda, MD, 2008, American Society of Health-System Pharmacists.

4

Intravenous Solutions, Stability, and Incompatibilities

LEARNING
OBJECTIVES

1. Discuss common intravenous fluids, including the abbreviations used.
2. Explain visual inspection of a parenteral solution.
3. List several factors that affect compatibility and stability of an intravenous solution.
4. Use reference materials to find incompatibility, compatibility, and storage information.

TERMS &
DEFINITIONS

Admixture The preparation of an intravenous (IV) medication that requires a mixture of medications

Clarity Clear and free of visible particulate matter

Compatibility Ability to combine drugs or substances without interfering with their action

Coring Breaking off small pieces of the rubber stopper on vials and allowing them to enter the solution or IV fluid

Hypertonic Any solution containing a higher concentration of dissolved substances than red blood cells

Hypotonic Any solution containing a concentration of dissolved substances less than red blood cells

Incompatibility Drugs and drugs, or drugs and fluids, that cannot be put together due to the incident of unwanted or unexpected effects

Isotonic Any solution containing a concentration of dissolved substances, such as salts, that are the same as the concentration found in human red blood cells

Osmolarity Number of dissolved particles in a solution per liter of solution

Osmosis Movement of a solvent (water) across a cell membrane from a lower osmolality to a higher osmolality

pH Degree of alkalinity or acidity of a solution. Acidity is usually between 0 to 6 while alkaline is between 8 to 14. Neutral pH is around 7.

Precipitation Solid material or deposits that are separated from a solution often caused from reactions between drugs or drugs and certain fluids

Reconstitution Process of adding a diluent to a powder form of a medication

INTRODUCTION

Errors can occur at any time, but when technicians prepare admixtures, chances are significantly increased due to the complexity of special procedures, equipment, and fluids that must be used. Often there is minimal supervision during the actual process, and this requires technicians to be even more conscientious about their technique and understanding of the medications that they are preparing. In this chapter, we will discuss common intravenous (IV) fluids, their industry abbreviations and their characteristics, compatibilities, and reference sources that are available for the technician to use.

Characteristics of Different Solutions Used in Intravenous Therapy

IV solutions used in parenteral administration must be prepared using aseptic technique and have certain characteristics. They must be sterile (that is, free from bacteria). They must also have *clarity,* which means clear and free of visible particulate matter. In addition to the clarity and being bacteria free, the solutions also have characteristics that determine how they will act once they are in the blood stream. *Osmosis* is the passage of water particles from an area of lower concentration to an area of higher concentration across a barrier, such as a cell membrane. The number of these dissolved particles per liter of solution is known as *osmolarity.* The *pH* of the solution is also very important because the body's fluid is slightly alkaline or about 7.4 (Figure 4-1).

Fluid entering the bloodstream that is too acidic or too alkaline can cause pain or discomfort, and damage to the red blood cells should be avoided if possible. The fluid inside the cell contains dissolved substances, such as sugars and salts. The cell membrane is designed to allow fluid to pass freely from one membrane to another but not the substances. *Isotonic* fluids have the same osmolarity as normal body fluid. These solutions are the closest to the red blood cells because the concentration of the salt and other substances are the same as those found in red blood cells. Both 5% dextrose and 0.9% sodium chloride are examples of isotonic fluids. If the solution contains a concentration of dissolved substances less than red blood cells, it is known as *hypotonic.* This means fluid will move into the cells and cause swelling. If the solution contains a higher concentration than the red blood cells, it is *hypertonic* and cells can shrink due the movement of fluids out of the cells. Both of these types of fluids can cause stinging because the cells are trying to either swell or shrink to handle the fluids introduced (Figure 4-2).

There are several common IV fluids available today. Medications that are added to the fluid are known as *additives,* whereas the final product is known as the *admixture.* Common IV fluids include sodium chloride injection, dextrose injection, and lactated Ringer's solution for injection (Figure 4-3). Dextrose injection (glucose) is primarily used as a carbohydrate for nutrition and as a source of fluid. It is usually given in 5% concentration. Sodium chloride is used as a source of fluid and electrolytes. It is usually given in 0.9%. Lactated Ringer's solution for injection contains primary electrolytes found in plasma and is used for fluid replacement or as a source of electrolytes.

All of these fluids can be found in various combinations and can also be manufactured with certain additives already in them. There are also standard abbreviations that are used when writing orders or prescriptions that technicians should be familiar with (Table 4-1).

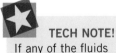

TECH NOTE!
If any of the fluids listed in Table 4-1 are manufactured with additives already added, the bag would have the additive written in red, such as dextrose 5% and 0.9% normal saline with 20 mEq of potassium chloride (D5NS20KCL).

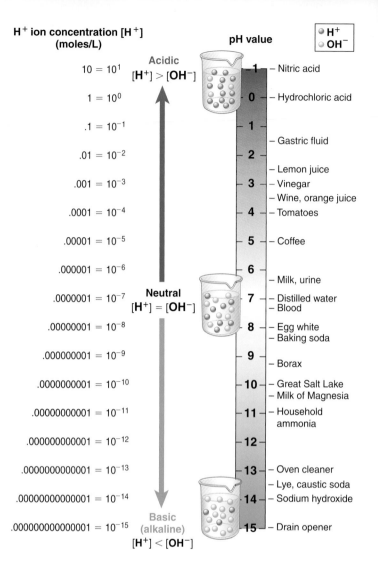

FIGURE 4-1 The pH scale. (From Patton KT, Thibodeau GA: *Anatomy & physiology*, ed 8, St Louis, 2012, Mosby Elsevier.)

H⁺ ion concentration [H⁺] (moles/L)

$10 = 10^1$	
$1 = 10^0$	
$.1 = 10^{-1}$	
$.01 = 10^{-2}$	
$.001 = 10^{-3}$	
$.0001 = 10^{-4}$	
$.00001 = 10^{-5}$	
$.000001 = 10^{-6}$	
$.0000001 = 10^{-7}$	
$.00000001 = 10^{-8}$	
$.000000001 = 10^{-9}$	
$.0000000001 = 10^{-10}$	
$.00000000001 = 10^{-11}$	
$.000000000001 = 10^{-12}$	
$.0000000000001 = 10^{-13}$	
$.00000000000001 = 10^{-14}$	
$.000000000000001 = 10^{-15}$	

Acidic
$[H^+] > [OH^-]$

Neutral
$[H^+] = [OH^-]$

Basic (alkaline)
$[H^+] < [OH^-]$

● H⁺
○ OH⁻

pH value

- −1 — Nitric acid
- 0 — Hydrochloric acid
- 1 —
- — Gastric fluid
- 2 —
- — Lemon juice
- 3 — Vinegar
- — Wine, orange juice
- 4 — Tomatoes
- 5 — Coffee
- 6 —
- — Milk, urine
- 7 — Distilled water
- — Blood
- 8 — Egg white
- — Baking soda
- 9 — Borax
- 10 — Great Salt Lake
- — Milk of Magnesia
- 11 — Household ammonia
- 12 —
- 13 — Oven cleaner
- — Lye, caustic soda
- 14 — Sodium hydroxide
- 15 — Drain opener

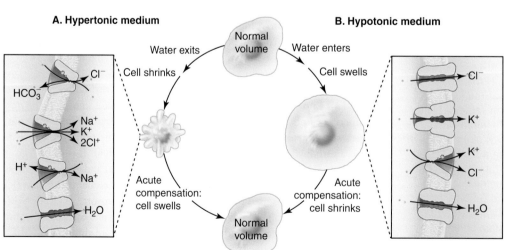

A. Hypertonic medium

Water exits
Cell shrinks

Cl⁻
HCO₃
Na⁺
K⁺
2Cl⁺
H⁺ → Na⁺
→ H₂O

Acute compensation: cell swells

Normal volume

Water enters
Cell swells

B. Hypotonic medium

Cl⁻
K⁺
K⁺
Cl⁻
→ H₂O

Acute compensation: cell shrinks

Normal volume

FIGURE 4-2 Cell behavior in hypotonic and hypertonic solutions. (From Pollard TD, Earnshaw WC: *Cell biology*, ed 2, Philadelphia, 2008, Saunders Elsevier.)

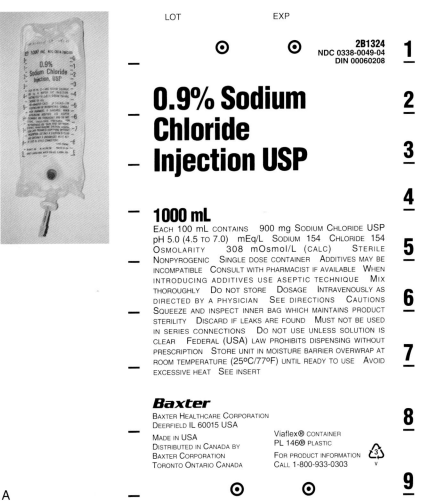

LOT   EXP

2B1324
NDC 0338-0049-04
DIN 00060208

1

0.9% Sodium Chloride Injection USP

2

3

4

1000 mL

EACH 100 mL CONTAINS   900 mg SODIUM CHLORIDE USP
pH 5.0 (4.5 TO 7.0) mEq/L SODIUM 154 CHLORIDE 154
OSMOLARITY   308 mOsmol/L (CALC)   STERILE
NONPYROGENIC SINGLE DOSE CONTAINER ADDITIVES MAY BE
INCOMPATIBLE CONSULT WITH PHARMACIST IF AVAILABLE WHEN
INTRODUCING ADDITIVES USE ASEPTIC TECHNIQUE   MIX
THOROUGHLY DO NOT STORE DOSAGE INTRAVENOUSLY AS
DIRECTED BY A PHYSICIAN SEE DIRECTIONS CAUTIONS
SQUEEZE AND INSPECT INNER BAG WHICH MAINTAINS PRODUCT
STERILITY DISCARD IF LEAKS ARE FOUND MUST NOT BE USED
IN SERIES CONNECTIONS DO NOT USE UNLESS SOLUTION IS
CLEAR FEDERAL (USA) LAW PROHIBITS DISPENSING WITHOUT
PRESCRIPTION STORE UNIT IN MOISTURE BARRIER OVERWRAP AT
ROOM TEMPERATURE (25ºC/77ºF) UNTIL READY TO USE AVOID
EXCESSIVE HEAT SEE INSERT

5

6

7

Baxter

BAXTER HEALTHCARE CORPORATION
DEERFIELD IL 60015 USA

MADE IN USA   Viaflex® CONTAINER
DISTRIBUTED IN CANADA BY   PL 146® PLASTIC
BAXTER CORPORATION   FOR PRODUCT INFORMATION
TORONTO ONTARIO CANADA   CALL 1-800-933-0303

8

9

A

FIGURE 4-3 Labels for sodium chloride **(A)**, dextrose **(B)**, and lactated Ringer's solution **(C)**. (From Brown M, Mulholland JL: *Drug calculations: process and problems for clinical practice,* ed 8, St Louis, 2007, Mosby Elsevier.)

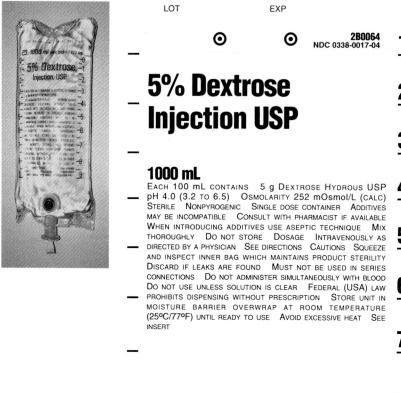

LOT   EXP

⊙   ⊙   **2B0064**
NDC 0338-0017-04

1

2

5% Dextrose Injection USP

3

1000 mL
EACH 100 mL CONTAINS   5 g DEXTROSE HYDROUS USP
pH 4.0 (3.2 TO 6.5)   OSMOLARITY 252 mOsmol/L (CALC)
STERILE NONPYROGENIC SINGLE DOSE CONTAINER ADDITIVES
MAY BE INCOMPATIBLE   CONSULT WITH PHARMACIST IF AVAILABLE
WHEN INTRODUCING ADDITIVES USE ASEPTIC TECHNIQUE   MIX
THOROUGHLY   DO NOT STORE   DOSAGE   INTRAVENOUSLY AS
DIRECTED BY A PHYSICIAN SEE DIRECTIONS CAUTIONS SQUEEZE
AND INSPECT INNER BAG WHICH MAINTAINS PRODUCT STERILITY
DISCARD IF LEAKS ARE FOUND   MUST NOT BE USED IN SERIES
CONNECTIONS   DO NOT ADMINISTER SIMULTANEOUSLY WITH BLOOD
DO NOT USE UNLESS SOLUTION IS CLEAR   FEDERAL (USA) LAW
PROHIBITS DISPENSING WITHOUT PRESCRIPTION   STORE UNIT IN
MOISTURE BARRIER OVERWRAP AT ROOM TEMPERATURE
(25ºC/77ºF) UNTIL READY TO USE   AVOID EXCESSIVE HEAT   SEE
INSERT

4

5

6

7

Baxter
BAXTER HEALTHCARE CORPORATION Viaflex® CONTAINER
DEERFIELD IL 60015 USA   PL 146® PLASTIC
MADE IN USA   FOR PRODUCT INFORMATION
                                CALL 1-800-933-0303

8

B   —   ⊙   ⊙   **9**

FIGURE 4-3, cont'd

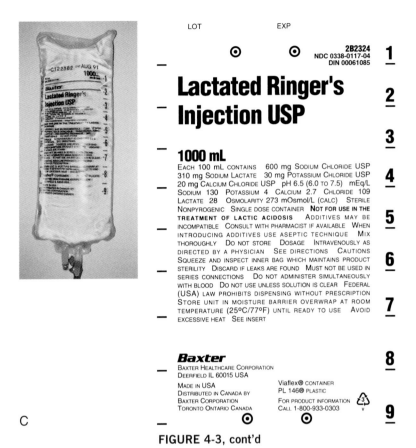

LOT   EXP

2B2324
NDC 0338-0117-04
DIN 00061085

1

Lactated Ringer's Injection USP

2

3

1000 mL

EACH 100 mL CONTAINS   600 mg SODIUM CHLORIDE USP
310 mg SODIUM LACTATE   30 mg POTASSIUM CHLORIDE USP
20 mg CALCIUM CHLORIDE USP   pH 6.5 (6.0 TO 7.5)   mEq/L
SODIUM 130   POTASSIUM 4   CALCIUM 2.7   CHLORIDE 109
LACTATE 28   OSMOLARITY 273 mOsmol/L (CALC)   STERILE
NONPYROGENIC   SINGLE DOSE CONTAINER   **NOT FOR USE IN THE
TREATMENT OF LACTIC ACIDOSIS**   ADDITIVES MAY BE
INCOMPATIBLE   CONSULT WITH PHARMACIST IF AVAILABLE   WHEN
INTRODUCING ADDITIVES USE ASEPTIC TECHNIQUE   MIX
THOROUGHLY   DO NOT STORE   DOSAGE   INTRAVENOUSLY AS
DIRECTED BY A PHYSICIAN   SEE DIRECTIONS   CAUTIONS
SQUEEZE AND INSPECT INNER BAG WHICH MAINTAINS PRODUCT
STERILITY   DISCARD IF LEAKS ARE FOUND   MUST NOT BE USED IN
SERIES CONNECTIONS   DO NOT ADMINISTER SIMULTANEOUSLY
WITH BLOOD   DO NOT USE UNLESS SOLUTION IS CLEAR   FEDERAL
(USA) LAW PROHIBITS DISPENSING WITHOUT PRESCRIPTION
STORE UNIT IN MOISTURE BARRIER OVERWRAP AT ROOM
TEMPERATURE (25°C/77°F) UNTIL READY TO USE   AVOID
EXCESSIVE HEAT   SEE INSERT

4

5

6

7

Baxter
BAXTER HEALTHCARE CORPORATION
DEERFIELD IL 60015 USA
MADE IN USA
DISTRIBUTED IN CANADA BY
BAXTER CORPORATION
TORONTO ONTARIO CANADA

Viaflex® CONTAINER
PL 146® PLASTIC
FOR PRODUCT INFORMATION
CALL 1-800-933-0303

8

9

C

FIGURE 4-3, cont'd

TABLE 4-1   **Standard Abbreviations and Tonicity of Intravenous Solutions**

IV Solution	Abbreviation	Tonicity
5% Dextrose	D5W	Isotonic
0.9% Sodium chloride	NS (normal saline)	Isotonic
Lactated Ringer's solution	LR	Isotonic
10% Dextrose	D10W	Hypertonic
0.45% Sodium chloride (normal saline)	1/2NS	Hypotonic
5% Dextrose and 0.9% sodium chloride	D5NS	Hypertonic
5% Dextrose and 0.45% sodium chloride	D51/2NS	Hypertonic
5% Dextrose and 0.2% sodium chloride	D51/4NS	Isotonic
Lactated Ringer's solution and 5% dextrose	D5LR	Hypertonic

Compatibility and Incompatibility of Intravenous Fluids

When combining medications in IV fluids, the ***compatibility*** of the admixture must be considered. Often there are drugs that cannot be combined safely with a particular IV fluid for various reasons. There may be a physical change (such as color or clarity) or a formation of particles called *particulate matter*. These IV admixtures are known as ***incompatible*** and must not be given to the patient. When preparing IV admixtures, carefully inspect the completed product visually, and look for any obvious changes. Any leaks, tears, or changes in the bag of fluid should be observed while still in the hood.

Look for the following characteristics:
- Particles floating, such as rubber from the stopper of the vial (known as ***coring***)
- Any color changes
- Haze or turbidity
- Solid particles or filaments formed (particulate matter)

Some incompatibilities cannot be seen with visual inspection but are just as important. These factors can affect the compatibility and/or stability of the drugs in an IV admixture, and reference materials, such as package inserts or Trissel's *Handbook on Injectable Drugs,* will provide storage and compatibility information about each drug specifically.

Some of these factors are discussed in the following sections.

TECH NOTE!
Always refer to medication information concerning compatibility. Color changes or particulate matter does not always form immediately. It may take hours for this to happen, and in that amount of time, the IV may be delivered to the patient for administration.

TEMPERATURE

Drugs often degrade due to storage in improper temperatures. Some drugs must be refrigerated, some kept at room temperature, and some may even be frozen for storage. For example, metronidazole (Flagyl) should be kept at room temperature because refrigeration causes precipitate to form.

LIGHT

Some drugs must not be exposed to light and should be protected by a light-blocking protective bag or cover because the medication will be destroyed or degraded. Often, vials of medication are packaged in colored or tinted containers to protect them. During administration, the admixture is protected from light by using special brown bags that block the light.

TIME

Once medications are added to an IV fluid, the amount of time that they are stable may change from the manufacturer's information provided in the packaging. This is because the drug has been taken from its original packaging and added to a sterile solution, which changes how it reacts with that fluid.

For instance, once a vial of cefazolin is reconstituted and added to a bag of 0.9% sodium chloride, the admixture is only good for 7 days at 4°C in its original vial, it would be good for years.

DILUTION

Medications can often be added to an IV fluid in certain concentrations and be compatible, but they will produce participates if they are added in higher concentrations. For example, when mixing calcium and phosphates, only 15 mEq of calcium can be added to a liter of fluid containing 30 mEq of phosphate without precipitating.

COMPATIBILITY

Some drugs will interact with certain metals, such as cisplatin (a chemotherapy drug) and aluminum. There are also medications that interact with PVC plastic, and contact between them should be avoided.

pH

If the fluid and medication to be added have conflicting pH values, this may cause the drug to either degrade or form a precipitate. An example is ampicillin, which is an antibiotic that has a pH of 8 to 10 as packaged in a vial from the manufacturer. As an admixture, the fluid of choice is sodium chloride 0.9%. Sodium chloride is preferred over dextrose because of the decomposition of the drug when mixed in dextrose during clinical studies.

INTRAVENOUS SOLUTION

Some drugs are only compatible with certain IV fluids, and the reference materials will indicate this. For example, ampicillin cannot be mixed in lactated Ringer's solution because the ampicillin will degrade within about 24 hours. However, when ampicillin is mixed with sodium chloride (as recommended by the manufacturer's instructions), it is stable for 8 hours at room temperature. Other drugs cannot be added to the same IV fluid at the same time, such as furosemide and chlorpromazine, because ***precipitation*** will occur immediately.

ORDER OF MIXING

Some drugs can be mixed together only if they are mixed well in the fluid before the next additive is mixed. If they are given the opportunity to be diluted individually before immediately adding the next drug, then the chance of them coming in direct contact with each other will be decreased and allow them to be added to the same fluid.

Sources of Information and References Available

Once the order for an IV admixture is written, the next step for the technician is to verify that the components can be safely mixed, and if so, what concentrations they should be and in what order if any. Certain medications come in powder form and are to be diluted with certain fluids according to the manufacturer (Table 4-2).

Once the medication is diluted if necessary, the next step is choosing a proper IV solution that the medication can be added to. This can be found in literature, such as the package insert, Trissel's *Handbook on Injectable Drugs,* electronic databases, and incompatibility charts. Storage information can be found in these resources as well.

It is very important to label the final product with any storage information that is necessary, such as the expiration date, refrigeration if required, and any other special manufacturer's considerations. Whenever possible, avoid incompatibilities to ensure safe and effective patient care. For example:

- Always take the time to consult reference sources for information about the proper preparation required.
- Always be aware of special storage requirements.
- Always dilute with proper fluids according to the manufacturer's guidelines or literature.

DID YOU KNOW?
Some medications (such as intravenous immunoglobulin [IVIG], a plasma replacement therapy, and insulin, used for diabetes) cannot be shaken after ***reconstitution*** due to the excess foam that will develop.

TECH ALERT!
When in doubt about compatibility with drug-drug or drug-fluid, always refer to reference sources. Some incompatibilities do not always show up visually.

- Always double-check calculations.
- Always note any interactions with certain types of containers, such as plastic or aluminum.
- If the final product is not to be used immediately, it is best to refrigerate if appropriate.

A technician must always be aware of the medications and any special considerations concerning storage, mixing, and proper handling when performing aseptic technique. The patient's safety depends on it.

TABLE 4-2   **Example: Ceftriaxone Sodium (Rocephin)**

Vial Size	Volume of Diluent
For Intramuscular Use	
250 mg	0.9 mL
500 mg	1.8 mL
1 g	3.6 mL
2 g	7.2 mL
For Intermittent Intravenous Infusion	
250 mg	2.4 mL
500 mg	4.8 mL
1 g	9.6 mL
2 g	19.2 mL

REVIEW
QUESTIONS

1. List three possibilities for contamination of an injectable solution during the preparation.
2. Name a precaution that you think could prevent each of the above three possible contaminations that you listed.

CRITICAL
THINKING

For the following scenarios, use the most appropriate resource, and answer the questions:

1. A nurse calls the pharmacy and asks if she can add some morphine sulfate to a bag of heparin that is already hanging in the patient's room. Where can she find this information? Are these two drugs compatible with each other?
2. As a technician in an IV room, there is an order for ampicillin 1 gm stat to be given. Is it compatible with lactated Ringer's solution?
3. A nurse calls to ask if ceftazidime and ciprofloxacin are compatible.
4. The same nurse calls later and asks if heparin can be given with ciprofloxacin.

5. A nurse calls and states that she found a bag of ready-to-use metro-nidazole IV fluid on the counter in the nurse's office for a patient who has gone home. It was there when she left last night, and she wants to know if it can be credited and reused for another patient.

6. A technician is preparing an order for vancomycin on December 15, 2013, and finds one that has been credited in the refrigerator. It was made and dated December 10, 2013. Is this appropriate to reuse for this patient?

COMPETENCIES

INCOMPATIBILITIES, COMPATIBILITIES, AND STORAGE REQUIREMENTS FOR INTRAVENOUS MEDICATIONS

Evaluation Key: S= Satisfactory   NI= Needs Improvement

Name: Quarter: Date:

COMPETENCIES	STUDENT			INSTRUCTOR		
Student will be able to:	S	NI	Comments	S	NI	Comments
Describe visual incompatibilities, concentration effects, and pH.						
Discuss isotonic, hypotonic, and hypertonic fluids.						
Discuss common IV fluids and the abbreviations used.						
Describe particulate matter inspection.						
Explain how to perform visual inspection of a parenteral solution.						
List various reference materials and the type of information that they include pertaining to IV preparations.						
List several ways to avoid IV preparation incompatibilities.						

LAB ACTIVITY

For the following solutions or medications, use the resources provided to answer the questions:
1. What is the pH of premixed cimetidine HCL? How does it come (mg in solution)? If mixed with warfarin, describe what visual precipitate occurs.
2. Name two solutions that vancomycin can be mixed in. How long does the manufacturer state that it is good for when mixed with D5NS? If mixed with methotrexate, describe what precipitate occurs.
3. How is ceftriaxone (Rocephin) packaged? For intramuscular injection, how much diluent would you use for a 500 mg vial? If using SWFI and the concentration is 250 mg/mL, how long is it stable at 4°C? How long is the frozen premixed solution stable?
4. How is amphotericin B administered normally? Name any special considerations used when preparing an infusion. Name two solutions that are incompatible and describe what occurs.

Bibliography

1. Blanchard, Loeb. *Nurse's handbook of I.V. drugs,* ed 3, Burlington, MA, 2009, Jones & Bartlett.
2. Delgin JH, Vallerand AH. *Davis' drug guide for nurses,* ed 11, Philadelphia, 2009, F.A. Davis Company.
3. Gahart BL, Nazareno AR. *2008 Intravenous medications,* ed 24, St Louis, 2007, Mosby Elsevier.
4. Phillips L. *Manual of I.V. therapeutics: evidence-based practice for infusion therapy,* ed 5, Philadelphia, 2010, F.A. Davis Company.
5. Trissel LA. *Handbook on injectable drugs,* ed 15, Bethesda, MD, 2008, American Society of Health-System Pharmacists.
6. U.S. National Library of Medicine: *MedlinePlus: Drugs, Supplements, and Herbal Information* (website): http://www.nlm.nih.gov/medlineplus/druginformation.html. Accessed March 1, 2013.

5

Calculations Used in Intravenous Preparations

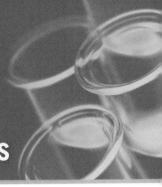

LEARNING OBJECTIVES

1. Calculate the volume of an injectable solution and the quantity of drug in an injectable solution.
2. Calculate powder volume for an injectable medication.
3. Calculate intravenous medications from a powder injectable.
4. Calculate intravenous flow rates for intravenous solutions.

TERMS & DEFINITIONS

Concentration Amount of medication per amount of fluid

Diluent Solution used to dilute a powder form of an injectable medication

Electrolytes Dissolved mineral salts, usually found in intravenous fluids, such as total parenteral nutrition or lactated Ringer's solution

Flow rate Amount of medication to be infused over a specific period of time

INTRODUCTION

When preparing intravenous (IV) admixtures, technicians must not only be careful to observe aseptic technique procedures but also be extremely cautious when calculating amounts of medications. These calculations are performed by pharmacists and technicians when the product is being prepared, as well as by the nurses who administer them. Special consideration should be taken with IV calculations since this route of administration bypasses the alimentary canal and goes directly into the bloodstream. If an error occurs, there is no way to remove the medication from the blood and reverse the unwanted effects. In this chapter, we will discuss calculating medication dosages, as well as common units of measurements and IV flow rates.

Medications given intravenously require special calculations. An intramuscular (IM) injection is given into the skeletal muscle in an aqueous form, and drugs that are water-based are absorbed quickly. If given subcutaneously (Sub-Q), the medication goes into the fatty layers of tissue and is absorbed quickly. An IV medication is given into the vein. All of these routes of administration are most often ordered in milligrams, and these can be administered at home, in the hospital, or in the office.

Calculations Involving Injectable Medications

When calculating the volume of an injectable medication, ratio and proportion is the most common method used. Medication labels will indicate the amount of medication in each unit, such as mg/mL. This information can then be used to calculate the amount of drug needed according to the physician's order or prescription.

IV medications are most often supplied in vials and ampules, which are glass containers. The amount of medication in a particular volume of fluid, such as microgram (mcg), milligram (mg), or gram (g) of medication in each milliliter (mL), will be on the label as the concentration. This will be used to determine how much should be dissolved in the appropriate liquid, such as normal saline (NS) or dextrose. The medication label may also use amounts of medication either in mg, unit (U), milliequivalent (mEq), or millimolar (mM) in a particular volume of fluid. Units are used for vitamins and chemicals while mEq and mM are measurements for *electrolytes,* such as sodium and potassium and certain drugs. The physician's order will either state the amount of volume needed or the amount of medication needed. With the amount of drug in a specific amount of fluid (*concentration*), a ratio and proportion calculation can determine the correct amount of drug to be used.

EXAMPLE 1

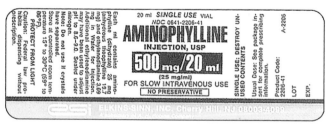

(From Ogden SJ, Fluharty L: *Calculation of drug dosages: a work text,* ed 9, St Louis, 2012, Elsevier Mosby.)

How many milliliters of aminophylline would be required to provide 1500 mg of medication?

$$\frac{500\,mg}{20\,mL} = \frac{1500\,mg}{X} \quad X\,mL = \frac{20\,mL \times 1500\,mg}{500\,mg} = 60\,mL$$

The ratio and proportion method can also be used to determine the amount of drug in an injectable solution.

EXAMPLE 2

NDC 0002-1675-01
20 mL   VIAL No. 419
℞
POISON   *Lilly*

ATROPINE
SULFATE
INJECTION, USP
0.4 mg
per mL
CAUTION—Federal (U.S.A.) law
prohibits dispensing without
prescription.

Store at 59° to 86°F (15° to 30°C)
Usual Adult Dose—0.75 to 1.5 mL injected
subcutaneously, intramuscularly, or slowly
intravenously. See literature.
Each mL contains Atropine Sulfate, 0.4 mg
with Chlorobutanol (Chloroform Derivative)
0.5 percent.
YA 9506 AMX
Eli Lilly & Co., Indianapolis, IN 46285, U.S.A.

APPROXIMATE EQUIVALENTS
0.4   mL = 0.16 mg
0.5   mL = 0.2 mg
0.6   mL = 0.24 mg
0.8   mL = 0.32 mg
1   mL = 0.4 mg
1.25 mL = 0.5 mg
1.6   mL = 0.65 mg
2.5   mL = 1.0 mg
3.1   mL = 1.25 mg

Exp. Date/Control No.

(From Ogden SJ, Fluharty L: *Calculation of drug dosages: a work text,* ed 9, St Louis, 2012, Elsevier Mosby.)

How many milligrams are in 3 mL of atropine?

$$\frac{0.4\,mg}{1\,mL} = \frac{X}{3\,mL}\ X\,mg = \frac{3\,mL \times 0.4\,mg}{1\,mL} = 1.2\,mg/3\,mL$$

Let's look at some typical IV orders that involve units such as insulin and heparin:
1. Order for heparin 12,000 units in NS 500 mL q8h. How many milliliters of heparin will be needed to prepare one bag?
   a. Choose the stock vial with the concentration of medication as close as possible to the desired concentration ordered (Figure 5-1). Since there are 10,000 units

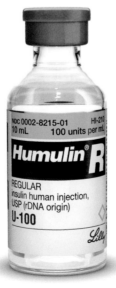

NDC 0002-8215-01   HI-210
10 mL   100 units per mL

Humulin®**R**

REGULAR
insulin human injection,
USP (rDNA origin)
U-100
Lilly

FIGURE 5-1 Insulin vial and label. (Courtesy Eli Lilly and Company, Indianapolis, IN)

in each milliliter of the stock vial of medication, this would be the most appropriate, because the order calls for just a little over 10,000 units of medication to be used.

b. $\dfrac{10{,}000\,\text{units}}{1\,\text{mL}} = \dfrac{12{,}000\,\text{units}}{X\,\text{mL}} \quad X\,\text{mL} = \dfrac{1\,\text{mL} \times 12{,}000\,\text{units}}{10{,}000\,\text{units}} = 1.2\,\text{mL of heparin}$

2. An order reads, "Add 44 mEq of sodium chloride (NaCl) to an IV bag." How many milliliters of sodium chloride will be needed for this order?

$$\dfrac{4\,\text{mEq}}{1\,\text{mL}} = \dfrac{44\,\text{mEq}}{X\,\text{mL}} \quad X\,\text{mL} = \dfrac{44\,\text{mEq} \times 1\,\text{mL}}{4\,\text{mEq}} = 1\,\text{mL}$$

Special Considerations for Parenteral Medications

POWDER VOLUME

Vials of medication can contain either a solution or a powder (Figure 5-2). If it is in powder form, it is made in a freeze-dried state and then placed in a sterile container. In order to create a solution from this and be able to draw up the contents in a syringe, the powder must be reconstituted by adding a solution, such as bacteriostatic water, sterile water, or saline, known as a **diluent.** The correct type and amount of diluent can be found in drug references, such as the package insert or the *Handbook on Injectable Drugs* by Trissell.[9] It is very important to use the manufacturer's recommended solution to dilute the powder because each drug and patient is different.

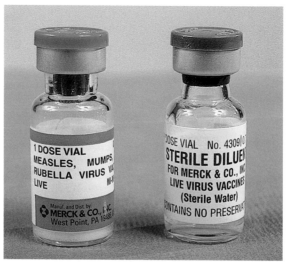

FIGURE 5-2 Vials, powdered form. (From Bonewit-West K: *Clinical procedures for medical assistants,* ed 8, St Louis, 2012, Elsevier Saunders.)

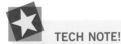

TECH NOTE!
Bacteriostatic water for injection USP is a nonpyogenic preparation of water injection containing 0.9% of benzyl alcohol as a bacteriostatic preservative (www.drugs.com).[3]
Since benzyl alcohol is toxic in neonates, it cannot be used as a diluent for IV dilution in this population.

This space that the powder occupies is known as *powder volume (PV)*. It is equal to the difference between the final volume (FV) and the volume of the diluting agent.

Formula

$$\text{powder volume (PV)} = \text{final volume (FV)} - \text{diluent volume (DV)}$$

EXAMPLE 3
A powder antibiotic known as nafcillin sodium needs to be reconstituted for use. You must follow the manufacturer's reconstitution directions and then prepare an IV bag.
1. How much diluent will be used? **6.6 mL**
2. What will the resulting powder volume be? *8 mL (FV) − 6.6 mL (DV)* = **1.4 mL (PV)**
3. What is the amount of medication in each milliliter? **250 mg**

EXAMPLE 4
You have an order for a medication that requires you to reconstitute 1 g of a dry powder. The label states to add 9.3 mL of diluent to make a final solution of 100 mg/mL. What is the powder volume?
   Step 1. Calculate the final volume by starting with the fact that 1 g is the same as 1000 mg of powder. Using the information, calculate the final volume using the ratio and proportion method:

$$\frac{1000\,\text{mg of powder}}{X\,\text{mL}} = \frac{100\,\text{mg}}{1\,\text{mL}} = 10\,\text{mL (FV)}$$

   Step 2. Using the **calculated** final volume, use the formula to determine the powder volume.

   Remember: powder volume (PV) = final volume (FV) − diluent volume (DV)

$$pv = 10\,\text{mL} - 9.3\,\text{mL} = 0.7\,\text{mL}$$

Calculation Examples for Intravenous Mixtures

PREPARING INTRAVENOUS MEDICATIONS FROM A POWDER INJECTABLE

EXAMPLE 5
Miss Davis has penicillin (Pfizerpen) 400,000 units/NS 100 mL ordered for a severe infection. After reading the dilution directions, you add 75 mL of diluent to the powder vial. Based on this information, how many milliliters will need to be added to the bag of NS 100 mL for the order?
   250,000 units in each milliliter is the amount of drug in each milliliter according to the label if 75 mL of diluent was added.

$$\frac{250,000\,\text{units}}{1\,\text{mL}} = \frac{400,000\,\text{units}}{X\,\text{mL}} = 250,000\,\text{units} \times X\,\text{mL}\ 400,000\,\text{units} \times 1\,\text{mL} = 1.6$$

The technician will now draw up 1.6 mL of Pfizerpen and add it to the bag of normal saline 100 mL.

EXAMPLE 6

Using the same medication as above, add 11.5 mL of diluent to the vial of penicillin (Pfizerpen), and answer the following questions concerning the following order for Mr. Brown:

Pfizerpen 6,000,000 in NS 100 mL STAT

1. How many units of medication is in each milliliter if 11.5 mL of diluent was added?
   Answer: 1,000,000 units/mL
2. How many milliliters of Pfizerpen will need to be added to the bag for a dose of 6,000,000 units?
   Answer:

$$\frac{1,000,000\ units}{1\ mL} = \frac{6,000,000\ units}{X\ mL} = 6\ mL$$

CALCULATING INTRAVENOUS ADMIXTURE FLOW RATES

An IV admixture order contains the IV fluid to be given, any additives, and the rate at which it should be infused. This **flow rate** is written as the amount of drug that is infused over a time period. This could be written as milliliters per hour (mL/hr) or drops per minute (gtt/min). Administration sets come in a variety of sizes and are measured by a drop factor. This is the number of drops in a milliliter. Often the order will require the drug to be administered with a pump or IV infusion set for drops per minute (gtt/min). The appropriate amount of medication must be given over a certain period of time to ensure that the therapeutic response is achieved. As a pharmacy technician, there are often times that you will have to determine how many bags to make in a batch in order to last 24 hours.

EXAMPLE 7

517410	
05/04/55	
K. Davis	DX: dehydration
Rm: 433	ALLERGIES: NKA
08/11/13	
1 L D5W with 20 mEq KCL added at 125 mL/hr	

NKA, No known allergies.

In the above example, this bag will last 8 hours.

$$time\ the\ bag\ will\ last = \frac{volume\ of\ fluid}{flow\ rate}$$

$$1 \text{ liter} = 1000 \text{ mL} \ \frac{1000 \text{ mL}}{125 \text{ mL} / \text{hr}} = 8 \text{ hours to infuse}$$

A new bag will be needed every 8 hours for this order. As a technician making a 24-hour supply of IV fluids for this patient, you would determine that three bags should be sent to the floor using the formula below:

$$\frac{24 \text{ hours}}{8 \text{ hours to infuse}} = 3 \text{ bags needed to last for 24 hours}$$

EXAMPLE 8
If an IV is running at 125 mL/hr and three 1 liter (L) bags are sent to the floor, how long will these bags last?

$$1 \text{ L} = 1000 \text{ mL} \times 3 = 3000 \text{ mL total volume}$$

$$X \text{ hr} = \frac{3000 \text{ mL (3 L)}}{125 \text{ mL/hr}} = 24 \text{ hours}$$

If the order specifies a certain amount of medication to be given over a specific time period, this can also be determined.

EXAMPLE 9
Medication: hydrocortisone sodium succinate (Solu-Cortef) 300 mg
Fluid volume: 250 mL
Time of infusion: 4 hours
What volume of fluid is to be given per hour, and what amount of drug is given per hour?
Determine the volume of fluid given by hour:

$$\frac{250 \text{ mL}}{4 \text{ hrs}} = 62.5 \text{ mL/hr}$$

The amount of drug per hour:

$$\frac{300 \text{ mg}}{4 \text{ hrs}} = 75 \text{ mg/hr}$$

Pumps are infusion devices, which are often used to deliver the IV therapy at home and in the hospital because they can ensure a predetermined flow rate. The amount of fluid can be programmed into the pump and then delivered to the patient safely (Figure 5-3).

Drop sets are used to manually adjust the flow at the drop chamber or set the IV pump at the patient's bedside (Figure 5-4). This setting can be determined by using mL/hr or gtts/mL, depending on the patient and the medication. The larger the diameter of the tubing where it enters the drip chamber, the bigger the drop will be. An IV set is identified by the number of drops it takes to make 1 mL.

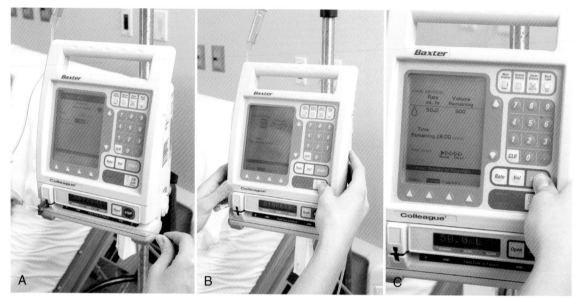

FIGURE 5-3 Baxter infusion pump. **A,** Insert IV tubing into chamber of control mechanism. **B,** Select rate and volume to be infused. **C,** Press start button. (From Perry AG, Potter PA, Elkin MK: *Nursing interventions and clinical skills,* ed 4, St. Louis, 2007, Elsevier Mosby.)

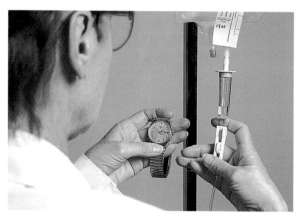

FIGURE 5-4 IV drop sets. (From Macklin D, Chernecky C, Infortuna MH: *Math for clinical practice,* ed 2, St Louis, 2011, Mosby Elsevier.)

Common sets include:
- 10 gtt/mL: Macro set commonly used for 125 mL/hr or more
- 15 to 20 gtt/mL: Macro set commonly used for 125 mL/hr
- 60 gtt/mL: Often referred to as the mini-drip or micro-drip set and generally used for delivering amounts of fluids per hour 50 mL/hr or less to critically ill or pediatric patients who are being given medication that is very specific in its dosing

To determine a flow rate using gtts/min, the following formula should be used.

$$X \, gtt/min = \frac{(\text{volume of fluid/delivery time}) \times (\text{set drop rate})}{60 \, min/hr}$$

EXAMPLE 10

If an IV is running at 60 mL/hr, what is the rate in gtt/min using a 15 gtt/mL set?
Volume of fluid: 60 mL
Fluid delivery time: 1 hour
Drop rate of administration set: 15 gtt/mL

$$X \, gtt/min = \frac{(60 \, mL/1hr) \times (15 \, gtt/mL)}{60 \, min/hr} = 15 \, gtt/min$$

EXAMPLE 11

You are to prepare an IV of 750 mg of medication in 75 mL to be infused over 30 minutes using a 10 gtt/mL set. How many drops per minute will that be?
Volume of fluid: 75 mL
Fluid delivery time: 30 minutes or 0.5 hours
Drop rate of administration set: 10 gtt/mL

$$X \, gtt/min = \frac{(75 \, mL/0.5 \, hr) \times (10 \, gtt/mL)}{60 \, min/hr} = 25 \, gtt/min$$

> **TECH ALERT!**
> Flow rates are rounded to the nearest whole gtt. This will ensure that the bag will not empty before the next one is hung.

When a micro-drip set is used, the flow rate in gtt/min is exactly the same as the volume in mL/hr to be infused because there are 60 minutes in an hour and 60 drops in a minute.

EXAMPLE 12

$$120 \, mL/hr \text{ using a micro-drip set} = 120 \, gtt/min$$

$$80 \, mL/hr \text{ using a micro-drip set} = 80 \, gtt/min$$

To determine the flow rate using gtt/mL, you must first determine the mL/hr that it is running. Then, convert that number to mL/min, and calculate the gtt/min.

EXAMPLE 13

An IV of 2500 mL is ordered to infuse in 24 hours using a 20 gtt/mL micro-drip set.

1. $\dfrac{2500 \, mL}{24 \, hrs} = 104 \, mL/hr$

2. $\dfrac{104 \, mL}{60 \, mins} = 1.7 \, mL/min$

3. $\dfrac{20 \, gtt}{1 \, mL} = \dfrac{X \, gtt}{1.7 \, mL} = 34 \, gtt/min$

A simpler way to show this is also included below:

$$\frac{(2500 \, \text{mL}/24 \, \text{hrs}) \times 20 \, \text{gtt}}{60 \, \text{min}} = 34.7 \text{ or } 34 \, \text{gtt}/\text{min}$$

Pain Controlled Analgesia

Often, patients require pain medications intravenously and medications, such as morphine, may be ordered to be infused by patient-controlled analgesia (PCA). PCAs are portable pumps designed for the patient to be able to give themselves a dose on demand.

EXAMPLE 14
The order would be written as follows:

Dr.

Address

Phone

DEA

For: _____

Address: _____ Date: _____

Morphine sulfate 1 mg every 10 minutes. Maximum dose is 30 mg in 4 hours.

☐ LABEL

REFILL _____ TIMES   _____

M.D.

The morphine concentration used is 1 mg/mL per 30-mL vial. What is the pump setting in mL/hr?

1 mg/10 minutes, 4-hour limit is 30 mg

EXAMPLE 15

```
┌─────────────────────────────────────────────────────────────────────┐
│  Dr.                                                                  │
│                                                                       │
│  Address                                                              │
│                                                                       │
│  Phone                                                                │
│                                                                       │
│  DEA                                                                  │
│                                                                       │
│                                                                       │
│  For: _____    │
│                                                                       │
│  Address:_____ Date:_____          │
│                                                                       │
│   ℞                                                                   │
│     Dilaudid 0.2 mg every 15 minutes. Maximum of 2 mg in 4 hours.     │
│                                                                       │
│                                                                       │
│                                                                       │
│                                                                       │
│  ☐ LABEL                                                              │
│                                                                       │
│  REFILL _____ TIMES          _____           │
│                                                                       │
│                                                           M.D.        │
└─────────────────────────────────────────────────────────────────────┘
```

The hydromorphone (Dilaudid) concentration is 1 mg/mL per 30-mL vial. What is the pump setting in mL/hr?

0.2 mg/15 minutes, 4-hour limit is 2 mg

Pediatric and elderly patients may need smaller volumes of fluids and medications than young adults. The physician may order the medication based on the recommended adult dose for milligrams per kilogram for 24 hours. Calculations will be determined by using the weight of the patient in kilograms.

Use the following formula:

mg/kg/day (24 hrs)

EXAMPLE 16

Ampicillin 900 mg intravenous piggyback (IVPB) q6h is ordered for a 75-pound patient. How many milligrams per kilogram per 24 hours is the patient receiving?

Convert pounds (lbs) to kilograms using the conversion of 1 kg = 2.2 lbs.

1. 1 kg = 2.2 lbs = x kg/75 lbs.
2. Cross multiply to get weight: 75 lb = 34.1 kg.

3. 900 mg × 4 doses = 3600 mg/24 hrs (24 hours divided by every 6 hours = 4 doses a day).
4. Calculate the dose using mg/kg/day:

$$\frac{(3600\,\text{mg/24 hrs})}{34.1\,\text{kg}} = 105.6\,\text{mg/kg/day}$$

5. The recommended dose is 100 to 200 mg/kg/day administered every 6 to 8 hours, so this would be an appropriate dose for this patient. Anything ordered between 100 to 200 mg/kg/day is within the range.

REVIEW QUESTIONS

1. The label of a 4 g vial states that you are to add 11.7 mL to get a concentration of 250 mg/mL. What is the powder volume?
2. The physician has ordered 2800 mL to be given every 24 hours. At what rate should the pump be set to in milliliters per hour?
3. If a patient is given 60 mg of medication in 75 mL over 45 minutes, what is the flow rate in mL/hr?
4. For the above problem, how many milligrams of medication will the patient receive?
5. An IV rate is set for 10 mL/hr. If a 10 gtt set is used, what will the rate be in gtt/min?

CRITICAL THINKING

1. A postoperative patient has an order for lactated Ringer's solution (LR) 1 L to be infused over 10 hours 3 days. How many milliliters per hour should the IV pump be programmed to deliver this order? How many bags should the technician prepare for a 24-hour period?
2. A pediatric patient has been ordered vancomycin 220 mg q6h IV using a syringe pump. He weighs 48 pounds, and the recommended manufacturer dosage is 40 to 60 mg/kg/24 hours q6h. How many mg/kg per 24 hours is the child receiving? Is this dose appropriate?

COMPETENCIES

CALCULATIONS USED IN INJECTABLE
MEDICATION PREPARATION

Evaluation Key: S= Satisfactory   NI= Needs Improvement

Name: _____   Quarter: _____   Date: _____

COMPETENCIES	STUDENT			INSTRUCTOR		
Student will be able to:	**S**	**NI**	**Comments**	**S**	**NI**	**Comments**
Interpret orders and required arithmetical calculations required for usual dosage determinations and solution preparations.						
Calculate IV drip rates and flow rates by various methods.						
Estimate and calculate time for IV administration.						
Calculate rates of infusion for IV solutions and piggybacks.						
Calculate the volume of an injectable solution.						
Calculate the powder volume for an IV solution.						
Calculate the quantity of drug in a given injectable solution.						

LAB ACTIVITY

Using the following order, calculate the concentration needed for the potassium chloride solution. Identify the solution needed in mEq/mL and the amount needed to draw up. Once calculations are completed, prepare the IV solution using proper aseptic technique.

Pt.name: John Doe	Room: 324	Date:

Potassium Chloride 25 mEq

Normal Saline 0.9% 1000 mls

Rate: 100 mls/hr

Keep refrigerated, expires in 24 hours.

Bibliography

1. Ballington DA, Green TW. *Pharmacy calculations for technicians,* ed 3, St. Paul, MN, 2007, EMC Paradigm Publishing.
2. Curren AM. *Math for meds: dosages & solutions,* ed 10, New York, 2008, Delmar Cengage Learning.
3. 2000-2013 Drugs.com: *Drug information online* (website): www.drugs.com. Accessed April 9, 2013.
4. Lacher, BE. *Pharmaceutical calculations for the pharmacy technician,* Baltimore, MD, 2008 Lippincott Williams & Wilkins.
5. Ogden SJ, Fluharty L. *Calculation of drug dosages: a work text,* ed 9, St Louis, 2012, Elsevier Mosby.
6. *Pediatric Medication Administration: Principles and Calculations,* New York, NY, 2003, Concept Media/Cengage Learning.
7. Pickar GD, Abernethy AP. *Dosage calculations,* ed 9, Clifton Park, NY, Delmar Cengage Learning.
8. Powers MF, Wakelin JB. *Pharmacy calculations,* ed 2, Englewood, CO, 2005, Morton Publishing Company.
9. Trissel LA. *Handbook on injectable drugs,* ed 15, Bethesda, MD, 2008, American Society of Health-System Pharmacists.

6

Equipment and Facilities

LEARNING OBJECTIVES

1. Discuss USP 797 guidelines and their importance in preventing microbial contamination.
2. Discuss requirements for the intravenous area according to USP 797, and demonstrate environmental procedures, including laminar air flow hood cleaning and proper garbing techniques.
3. Identify supplies used in aseptic technique, including how to read syringes.

TERMS & DEFINITIONS

Ante area International Organization for Standardization (ISO) Class 8 area where personal hand hygiene, garbing, and staging of components, order entry, labeling, and high particulate activities are performed before entering the buffer area

Biological safety cabinet (BSC) Special hood where air flows downward through a HEPA filter; used for chemotherapy preparation

Buffer area ISO Class 5 area where LAFW or other PECs are physically located and aseptic manipulations occur

Clean room Term sometimes used for *buffer area*

Contamination Introduction of pathogens or microbes into or on normally clean or sterile objects, surfaces, or spaces

Critical area ISO Class 5 environment where aseptic manipulations take place

Critical site Area to never touch (such as needle tips, tops of vials, and syringe plunger) to avoid cross contamination during aseptic manipulations

Direct compounding area (DCA) Area within the ISO Class 5 primary engineering control where manipulations are performed

First air Direct flow of air exiting the HEPA filter inside the DCA, which should never be interrupted and is essentially particle-free

Garbing Apparel or clothing that should be worn during aseptic preparation

Gauge (ga) Size of the needle shaft (thickness); the finer the needle, the higher the gauge number

High-efficiency particulate air (HEPA) filter Special filter used in the LAFW designed to remove 99.97% of particles that are 0.3 microns or larger. This creates a bacteria free environment to perform aseptic technique manipulations in.

Laminar airflow workbench (LAFW) Also known as the "hood." This area is designed to be used to perform aseptic technique in because it uses a HEPA filter to create an environment that produces sterile air.

61

Large volume parenteral (LVP) Containers of sterile solution used for intravenous medications; usually 500 mL to 3000 mL in volume

Personal protective equipment (PPE) Equipment, including shoe and hair covers, beard covers, gowns, masks, and gloves

Piggyback (PB) Containers of sterile solution used to administer medications through a secondary set or intermittent infusion; usually 50 mL to 250 mL in volume

Primary engineering control (PEC) Controls such as LAFWs, compounding aseptic isolators, or BSCs located in the buffer area

Secondary set When a piggyback infusion is hung higher than the main IV solution which allows it to run into the vein faster. An example would be an antibiotic that would be ordered to infuse in 30 minutes.

Small volume parenteral (SVP) Containers of sterile solutions used for intravenous medications; usually 50 mL to 100 mL or less in volume.

INTRODUCTION

Aseptic technique involves strict guidelines, and its primary goal is to prevent the spread of microbial contaminates. Technicians who prepare intravenous (IV) preparations must understand the importance of maintaining sterility and the importance of preventing medication errors. In order to safely prepare IV medications, the processes, guidelines, and proper handling of equipment is essential to avoid errors. In this chapter, we will discuss United States Pharmacopoeia Chapter 797 (USP 797) guidelines, aseptic technique, and the equipment and facilities that are used. We will also discuss the cleaning and proper *garbing* that is associated with this important task.

Aseptic Technique and USP 797 Guidelines Used in Intravenous Therapy

As of January 1, 2004, pharmacies compounding sterile preparations have been required to monitor their facilities and processes to standards mandated by USP 797. According to the USP 797 practice standards, certain guidelines must be followed because IV preparations are most hazardous to patients when administered into body cavities, such as veins, eyes, and the central nervous system. This chapter was written by a group of health care professionals and outlines the equipment, procedures, training requirements, validation processes, and even the environment to be used. These standards, along with the American Society of Health-System Pharmacists (ASHP) guidelines and the National Coordinating Committee on Large Volume Parenterals (NCCLVP) guidelines of practice, are designed to describe the conditions and practices needed to process compounded sterile preparations (CSPs) that will prevent harm or even death to patients resulting from *contamination.*

Environment, Garbing, and Equipment Cleaning Procedures

The first step in preparing aseptic preparations is the environment itself. The space where sterile preparation takes place must be clean and free from contaminates. This working space is divided into three sections (Figure 6-1).

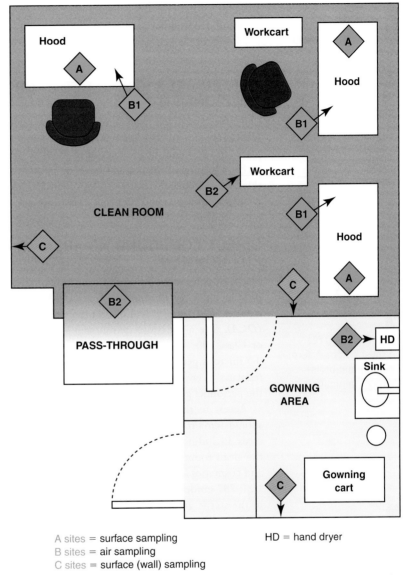

A sites = surface sampling
B sites = air sampling
C sites = surface (wall) sampling

HD = hand dryer

FIGURE 6-1 The layout of a buffer area (clean room). (Courtesy of CriticalPoint, LLC, Gaithersburg, MD.)

ANTE ROOM OR ISO CLASS 8 ENVIRONMENT

The ante room, or ISO Class 8 environment, is the outermost ring of the three areas. USP 797 defines this environment as the area where handwashing, garbing, gathering of components needed, order entry, labeling, and other activities that may "stir up dust." This area is located directly outside of the **buffer area,** where the handwashing and garbing procedure should be performed. The air in this room, or area, is considered an ISO Class 8 environment, which means that the air contains

100,000 particles of 0.5 microns per cubic meter or less. Cartons and packaged compounded supplies (such as needles, syringes, IV bags, and tubing sets) should be unpacked and wiped down with sterile 70% alcohol before passing on to the buffer area when possible.

BUFFER AREA (CLEAN ROOM) OR ISO CLASS 7 ENVIRONMENT

The buffer area is the main compounding area where *primary engineering controls (PECs)* are located. This room is where the actual aseptic manipulations of CSPs take place, and it should be located out of the flow of traffic and have limited personnel access. Opening of cartons and boxes or supplies should take place prior to entering this area to reduce the amount of dust particles and ensure a clean product. The buffer area is known as an ISO Class 7 environment, which means that the air contains no more than 10,000 particles of 0.5 microns per cubic meter or less.

DIRECT COMPOUNDING AREA OR ISO CLASS 5 ENVIRONMENT

The most common types of PECs are horizontal or vertical flow hoods. This *critical area* includes the *laminar airflow workbench (LAFW)* and the *biological safety cabinet (BSC),* and it is also commonly referred to as the *direct compounding area (DCA).* The air in this environment is considered an ISO Class 5 environment, or Class 100. This indicates that the air contains no more than 100 particles of 0.5 microns per cubic meter or less. The microorganisms in this area are monitored regularly to ensure that the level of contaminates in the air, on the surfaces, and on the personnel gear do not exceed the specified cleanliness class.

Access to the IV areas should be limited to only essential personnel. Doors should remain closed at all times, and no food or drink is ever allowed in these areas, including gum chewing! Avoid coughing, sneezing, and excessive talking in the clean room to avoid adding any additional contaminates to the area. Jewelry and cosmetics are restricted upon entry into the ante area according to the current USP 797 guidelines. Artificial nails or extenders are also prohibited while working in the sterile area, and fingernails should be natural and kept trimmed and neat. Additionally, no shipping or external cartons should ever be in the buffer area (also known as the *clean room*).

LAMINAR AIRFLOW WORKBENCH AND BIOLOGICAL SAFETY CABINET

The LAFW or BSC are both areas that provide a Class 5 environment for aseptic preparation inside the buffer area (Figure 6-2).

LAFWs should be placed out of the traffic flow and are the cleanest work surface in the system. The most important part of this "hood," as it is sometimes referred to, is the special filter known as a *high-efficiency particulate air (HEPA) filter.* The filter should never be touched, cleaned, or sprayed with alcohol.

Sitting in front of the LAFW is like sitting in front of a fan blowing wind in your face. The air, known as *critical air,* enters the prefilter at the front of the hood, travels through the HEPA filter at the back where bacteria and other air contaminants are removed, and then flows horizontally across the work surface (Figure 6-3). This allows purified air to circulate from the back to the front constantly in parallel lines. The air

Vertical Hood

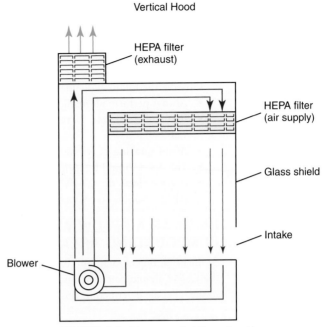

FIGURE 6-2 Diagram of airflow direction.

Horizontal Hood

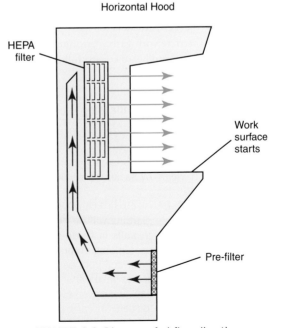

FIGURE 6-3 Diagram of airflow direction.

space inside the LAFW is the area known as the DCA. This is where exposure to HEPA-filtered air, or *first air*, occurs when preparing aseptic preparations. ***Critical sites*** (such as the tops of vials and needle surfaces) should always be exposed to first air to avoid contamination from particles allowed to linger in the air. Surfaces (such as needles, syringe plungers, or vial tops) should be exposed to first air at all times.

Observe the following guidelines when working in the LAFW:

- Always perform all manipulations at least 6 inches inside the hood.
- Remember first air: Never interrupt the airflow between the HEPA filter and sterile objects.
- Avoid spraying or wiping the HEPA filter.
- The hood should be turned on at least 30 minutes prior to using.
- Always clean the LAFW with an approved agent (70% isopropyl alcohol [IPA]) and lint-free wipes.

LAMINAR AIRFLOW WORKBENCH (HOOD) OR DIRECT COMPOUNDING AREA CLEANING PROCEDURE

At the beginning of each shift, before a batch, after spills, and at least every 30 minutes, the LAFW should be cleaned using the procedure outlined in Box 6-1 and according to the schedule described in Box 6-2.

GARBING

USP 797 also has specific guidelines for the apparel or clothing that should be worn during aseptic manipulations as well as a certain order for donning ***personal protective equipment (PPE),*** such as gloves, gowns, and hair covers. PPE is designed to prevent the spread of infectious diseases during aseptic preparation (Figure 6-4).

Before entering the ante room, personnel shall remove outer garments (such as jackets, sweaters, or hats), all cosmetics, and any visible jewelry or piercings that interfere with garb. Personnel should don garb beginning with shoe covers, then hair nets and beard covers, followed by face shields or masks. In general, the order should

BOX 6-1   **Cleaning Procedure of the Laminar Airflow Workbench**

SUPPLIES FOR CLEANING THE LAFW
Lint free cloth
Sterile 70% isopropyl alcohol (IPA)
Begin by soaking a stack of cloths with the alcohol.

CLEAN IN THE FOLLOWING ORDER
(*Note:* Garbing will be performed prior to any cleaning activities.)
1. Clean walls in an up-and-down motion working outward from back to front.
2. Use automated compounders (if necessary).
3. Work surface from back to front in long strokes. Start at the back corner, and go across in parallel lines working your way to the front being careful to overlap and cover every area of the work surface. As the stack of cloths get dirtied, discard them. Allow the area to dry before beginning aseptic manipulations. *Note:* Be sure to overlap slightly when wiping to prevent any areas of the surface from being missed.

BOX 6-2   **Cleaning Schedule for the Laminar Airflow Workbench**

DAILY SCHEDULE

Floors, counters, and easily cleanable work surfaces in the ante area and buffer area should be cleaned and disinfected daily when no aseptic operations are in progress. This includes the sink and all contact surfaces.

Supplies Needed for Cleaning
- Disinfectant solution, such as diluted bleach
- Microfiber cleaning system (alternative to mop)

Cleaning Techniques
- Clean all counters and cleanable work surfaces with disinfectant.
- Mop the floor, starting at the wall opposite of the room entry door.
- Mop in even strokes toward the operator, moving carts as needed.
- In the ante room, clean the sink and contact surfaces, and clean the floor as described above.

MONTHLY SCHEDULE

Wall, storage shelving, and ceilings should be cleaned and disinfected monthly with a germicidal detergent-soaked, lint-free wipe and then followed with 70% IPA. This includes wiping the inside of trash cans, emptying storage bins, and cleaning chairs in the buffer area.

Document all cleaning procedures; include who performed the activities along with dates and times, and include these records as part of the quality assurance program for the facility.

TECH NOTE!
If the gloves become contaminated by touching a non-sterile surface, you can reapply 70% alcohol to the surface area of the gloves and let dry thoroughly.

be dirtiest to cleanest (for example, shoe covers before head covers). Hospitals may have slight variations for this procedure due to room layout and facility protocols.

Perform hand cleansing (see the handwashing procedure described in Chapter 1). Don a non-shedding gown that fits snugly around the wrists and neck. Upon entering the buffer area, perform antiseptic hand cleansing with antiseptic waterless alcohol-based surgical hand scrub, and then don sterile gloves. Remember, no food, drinks, candy, gum, or unnecessary items are allowed in the buffer area. Only compounding personnel should be in this area.

When exiting the buffer area, the gown may be reused during the same work shift if it remains in the buffer area and is not soiled. However, shoe covers, masks, and gloves need to be replaced, and handwashing needs to be performed if the buffer area is re-entered.

In addition, only stainless steel shelving and nonporous surfaces are allowed in the ISO Class 7 environment (buffer area) where the PECs are located. Items such as computers, carts, and nonessential containers should not be stored or kept in this room. Staging of items and calculations should take place before entering the LAFW (clean room), and only immediate need items, not cases of fluids, should be in this room because cardboard will cause excessive dust and contamination. Sampling the air quality in the ISO Classes 5, 7, and 8 should be tested no less than every 6 months.

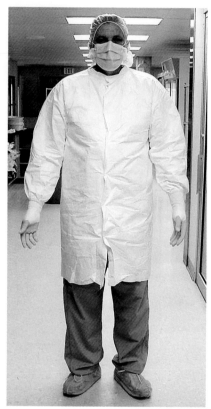

FIGURE 6-4 A technician in full personal protective equipment (PPE). (Courtesy of CriticalPoint, LLC, Gaithersburg, MD.)

Supplies Used in Aseptic Preparation

Supplies (such as syringes, needles, alcohol pads, solution containers, vials, ampules, and filters) are commonly used in IV preparations.

Syringes are used to draw up solutions or medications to be injected into a solution container. Sterile disposable syringes are packaged individually and should be discarded after one use. They consist of two parts: the barrel and the plunger (Figure 6-5).

The plunger is a piston-type rod that is cone-shaped on one end and is inside of the barrel of the syringe. The other end has flanges on it for hand placement. The barrel has graduations on it to indicate the volume of the solution held inside. Each size has its own graduations and varies from milliliters to fractions of milliliters. Insulin syringes known as U-100 (or 100 units per mL/cc) have units indicated on them as well as fractions of millimeters. This is because insulin orders are normally written as units, such as *50 units regular insulin qd* (Figure 6-6). When very small doses are required, they are measured in tuberculin (TB) syringes, which are calibrated in hundredths.

TECH ALERT!
The plunger, tops of vials, and the tip of a syringe are considered critical sites and should never be touched.

DID YOU KNOW?
A mL and a cc is the same measurement?

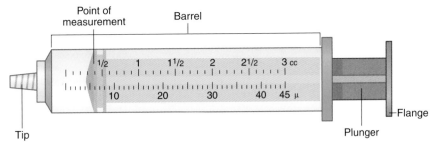

FIGURE 6-5 Anatomy of a syringe. (From Hopper T: *Mosby's pharmacy technician: principles and practice,* ed 3, St Louis, 2011, Elsevier Saunders.)

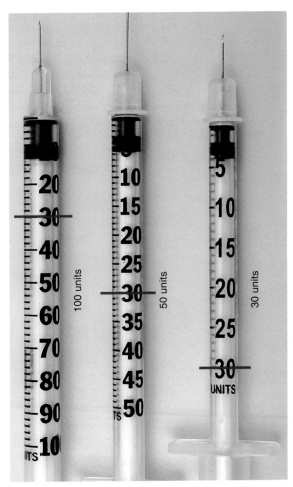

FIGURE 6-6 From left to right: 30 units measured on a 100-unit syringe (each calibration is 2 units), a 50-unit syringe (each calibration is 1 unit), and a 30-unit syringe (each calibration is 1 unit). (From Macklin D, Chernecky C, Infortuna MH: *Math for clinical practice,* ed 2, St Louis, 2011, Mosby Elsevier.)

For example:

60 cc	Each line indicates 1 mL or cc.
20 cc	Each line indicates 1 mL or cc.
10 cc or 12	Each line indicates 0.2 mL or cc or two-tenths.
5 cc or 6	Each line indicates 0.2 mL or cc or two-tenths.
3 cc	Each line indicates 0.1 mL or cc or tenths.
1 cc	Each line indicates 0.02 mL or cc or hundredths.
TB	Each line indicates 0.02 mL or cc or hundredths.
Insulin	Each line indicates 0.02 mL or cc or hundredths.

TECH ALERT!
Syringes and needles are most often disposable and should be discarded after one use. The tips or locking-end of a syringe is a critical site and should never be touched.

Needles consist of two basic parts: a shaft and a hub. The shaft or long hollow tube has a bevel on the end. The hub is where it attaches to the syringe. Hubs are often colored to indicate the ***gauge (ga),*** or size, of the needle and range from 27 ga, which is the smallest or finest, to 13 ga, which is the largest. They also come in different lengths ranging from ⅜ to 3½ inches (Figure 6-7). The needle is attached to the syringe securely by a locking device, such as Luer-Lok. This allows the needle to attach more securely, because it is a circular collar that requires a half turn to lock the needle to the syringe. The needle can then be inserted into a container or vial, and fluid is drawn up into the barrel of the syringe. There are also vented needles that are used mainly for reconstituting a powder form of a medication. This process will be discussed in Chapter 7.

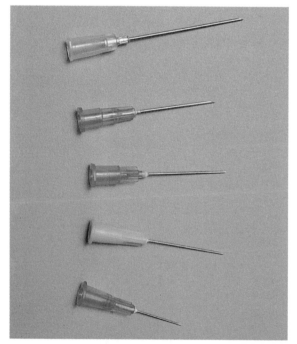

FIGURE 6-7 From top to bottom: Needle sizes shown are 19, 20, 21, 23, and 25 gauge. (From Hopper T: *Mosby's pharmacy technician: principles and practice,* ed 3, St Louis, 2011, Elsevier Saunders.)

Alcohol pads come in sterile packaging and should be used to wipe the tops of vials and other containers during sterile preparation (Figure 6-8). The proper way to use the pads is very important when cleaning a critical site, such as a vial top. The pad should only be used once by swabbing across the surface and allowed to dry completely before proceeding.

The process of the alcohol drying is when the dehydration of the bacteria cell occurs, which is necessary to kill it. If the alcohol is still "wet" during manipulations, it may allow microorganisms to be suspended in the fluid and cross over from one product to another during aseptic manipulations. In addition, 70% sterile IPA may be used to disinfect any work surfaces, ampule necks, vial tops, and IV injection ports on bags.

Vials are plastic- or glass-closed containers that hold medication in solution or powder form. They have a rubber stopper for the needle to be inserted and fluid to be withdrawn. Medication can also come in glass ampules, which are designed to be broken at the neck (Figure 6-9). Fluid is withdrawn using a special filter needle to catch all the glass particles that remain in the fluid. Once the fluid is withdrawn from the ampule into the syringe, the filter needle is removed and discarded, a new needle is placed on the syringe, and the contents can be injected into the bag.

Special filters are often required when preparing medication from an ampule or when particles must be removed from a solution. Filter straws may be used when withdrawing the contents of an ampule, but they are not needles. They can be replaced by a standard needle, added to the syringe, and used to add the medication to an IV bag via the port. These devices filter particles of varying sizes and attach on the end of the syringe, sometimes as a separate device or a special needle with the filtering mechanism inside of the hub itself. These filter needles can range in size from 0.22 microns to 10 microns, depending on the medication to be filtered.

Solution containers can vary in size and are usually plastic or glass. They have two ports on the end, one for adding medication with a needle and syringe and another to connect tubing. Bags from 50 mL to 250 mL are known as **_piggybacks (PBs)_** (Figure 6-10) or **_small volume parenterals (SVPs)_** and are generally used for

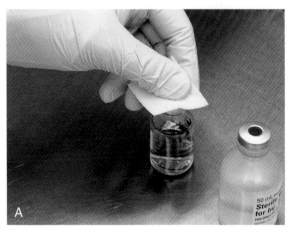
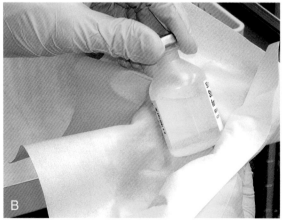

FIGURE 6-8 A, Wiping off the top of a vial (critical site area) with a sterile alcohol wipe, and **B,** Wiping the vial upon entry into the LAFW (hood area). (Courtesy of CriticalPoint, LLC, Gaithersburg, MD.)

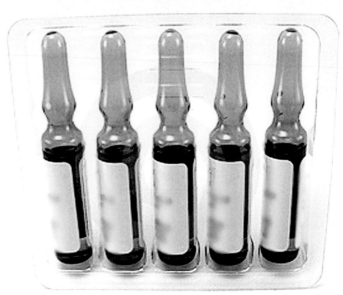

FIGURE 6-9 Ampules. (Courtesy of CriticalPoint, LLC, Gaithersburg, MD.)

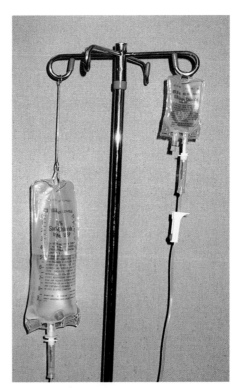

FIGURE 6-10 A set of piggybacks. (From Brown M, Mulholland JL: *Drug calculations: process and problems for clinical practice,* ed 8, St Louis, 2007, Mosby.)

antibiotics or small amounts of fluid. Bags from 500 mL to 1000 mL are known as *large volume parenterals (LVPs)* and can be used for fluid replacement and other types of medication therapy. There are also 2000 to 3000 mL bags used for total parenteral nutrition (TPN) or irrigation.

Tamper-evident seals are used to cover the port once a medication has been added to an IV bag. This indicates a medication has been added to a stock bag of fluid and ensures no breach of the sterile container prior to administration to the patient. Once the IV has been made, a label should be placed on the finished product to indicate the following:

- Name of patient
- Date prepared
- All solutions, ingredients, amounts, or concentrations
- Rate of infusion
- Storage requirements
- Expiration or beyond use date
- Name of preparer and checking pharmacist's initials
- Total volume and administration instructions

One of the most important aspects of aseptic technique is understanding the ways the environment ensures a sterile medication for the patient. Contamination can occur at many levels throughout the preparation of sterile medications, and technicians should be aware of the potential dangers in the process as well as the consequences of improper environmental controls. Along with proper training and equipment, the environment should be maintained and checked periodically according to UPS 797 standards by utilizing a quality assurance program. This will be discussed in Chapter 11.

REVIEW QUESTIONS

Identify the dosages measured on the following syringes by highlighting the measurement on the syringe.

1. 2.4 mL on a 3 cc syringe

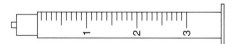

2. 10.6 mL on a 20 cc syringe

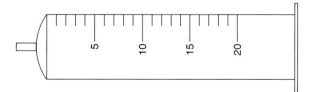

3. 30 U on a 1 cc insulin syringe

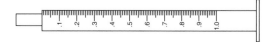

4. 10.4 mL on a 20 cc syringe

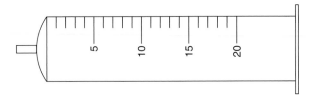

5. 12.5 cc on a 20 cc syringe

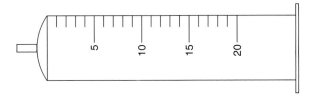

6. 1.5 cc on a 3 cc syringe

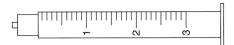

7. 0.06 mL on a TB syringe

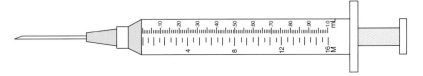

8. 0.15 cc on a TB syringe

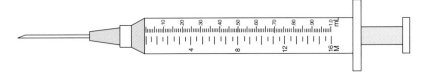

CRITICAL
THINKING

1. You are assigned to the IV room for the week, and you have a new externship student assigned to you. The student asks, "Is it really necessary to be so clean when preparing an antibiotic for a patient? Won't the medication kill any germs on the bag while it is fighting the patient's infection?" What would you say? Explain aseptic technique and why it is important to the patient.

2. Why is touch contamination the easiest form of contamination? Explain ways that using proper aseptic technique can prevent this from occurring.

COMPETENCIES

EQUIPMENT AND FACILITIES (USP 797) GUIDELINES FOR ASEPTIC COMPOUNDING

Evaluation Key: S = Satisfactory   NI = Needs Improvement

Name: _____   Quarter: _____   Date: _____

COMPETENCIES	STUDENT			INSTRUCTOR		
Student will be able to:	**S**	**NI**	**Comments**	**S**	**NI**	**Comments**
Define *aseptic techniques.*						
Discuss USP 797 and its primary goal.						
Identify common equipment used in aseptic compounding.						
Discuss environment and quality control for the aseptic compounding area.						
Identify common personal protective equipment (PPE) and why USP 797 garbing procedures are used.						
Explain cleaning procedures for the laminar airflow workbench (LAFW).						
List the common duties that can be performed in the ante area.						
List common duties performed in the buffer area.						
List several USP 797 guidelines to follow when working in the buffer area.						
Discuss the daily and monthly cleaning procedures for the aseptic compounding area.						
Discuss garbing procedures according to the USP 797 guidelines.						

LAB ACTIVITIES

Name: _____   Quarter: _____   Date: _____

PROCEDURE: GARBING	EVALUATION		
	Student	**Preceptor**	**Comments**
Ante Room			
Remove all cosmetics and jewelry.			
Nails are trimmed and natural.			
Don beard cover if required.			
Don hair cover or hairnet.			
Don face mask/eye shields.			
Don shoe covers.			
Perform handwashing. (Use Chapter 1 procedure check off.)			
Don a non-shedding gown.			
Buffer Area			
Use antiseptic hand cleanser.			
Don sterile gloves, and inspect for holes or tears. Reapply antiseptic hand cleaner over gloved hands.			
Document all cleaning procedures, including name and dates according to facility policy.			

Name: Quarter: Date:

PROCEDURE: CLEANING THE LAFW	EVALUATION		
	Student	Preceptor	Comments
Hood turned on at least 30 minutes prior			
Complete the garbing and handwashing procedures correctly as above.			
Use lint-free wipes and 70% IPA alcohol.			
Begin by soaking a stack of lint-free wipes.			
Clean walls from back to front, working outward in an up-and-down motion.			
Clean work surfaces from back to front in long strokes, going across from side to side.			
Start in back corner and go across in parallel lines, being careful to wipe every spot.			
Discard wipes in the stack as they become dirtied.			
Document procedures with name, date, and time according to facility policy.			

Bibliography

1. Pharmaceutical compounding-sterile preparations (general information chapter 797). In: The United States Pharmacopeia, 27th rev. and The National Formulary, 22nd ed. Rockville, MD: The United States Pharmacopeial Convention, 2004:2350-70.
2. Gahart BL, Nazareno AR. *2007 Intravenous medications*, ed 23, St Louis, 2007, Mosby.
3. Phillips LD: *Manual of I.V. therapeutics*, ed 4, Philadelphia, 2005, F.A. Davis Company.

7

Techniques for Preparing Intravenous Admixtures

TERMS & DEFINITIONS

Closed system Used to describe a vial which is a sealed container of solution where air is not allowed to move freely in and out of the container

Reconstitution Used to describe the process of adding a sterile solution to a vial of powdered medication in order to make a liquid

Stage Term used to describe how the final preparation is prepared for the pharmacist check of a sterile compound

Vented needle A specialty needle used when compounding with vials of powdered medications that require reconstitution

INTRODUCTION

Aseptic technique requires sterile equipment and a sterile environment, but it also includes manipulations that ensure sterility. Areas known as critical sites should never be touched in order to prevent contamination. These include tips of syringes, hubs of needles, ports of bags, tops of vials, and ends of filters or dispensing pins. Good hand placement will ensure the avoidance of contact to these areas as well as maintaining an open, direct path for first air in the laminar airflow workbench (LAFW) across these surfaces.

Before any manipulations can occur, certain tasks must be performed. Handwashing and garbing using the USP 797 guidelines are essential as well as cleaning the LAFW (see Chapter 6 for procedures). Technicians must understand these procedures and follow them in order to prevent contamination and subsequently avoid harm to the patient. We will discuss various techniques used in aseptic preparation, as well as manipulation of the equipment, in this chapter.

Aseptic technique is performed in the Class 5 environment, or clean room. Once proper handwashing and garbing is completed, the preparer begins the process of aseptic technique in the LAFW. The area where all aseptic manipulation takes place is the direct compounding area *(DCA).* Items are placed in the DCA one at a time by using a specific procedure.

First, only those items necessary should be placed in the DCA and excess paper items, such as alcohol pad paper and outer wrappers, are discarded on the outside. Each item used during aseptic manipulation, including syringes, needles, and medication vials, are sprayed with 70% isopropyl alcohol (IPA) and wiped down at the edge of the LAFW. Sterile supplies are removed from their outer wrappings at the edge of the DCA as they are introduced into the International Organization for Standardization (ISO) Class 5 area environment (LAFW, or biological safety cabinet [BSC]). All items are spread out at least 6 inches apart to ensure that there is sufficient space to work between them without disrupting the airflow or first air. In addition, items are kept at least 3 inches from the back and sides, and all manipulations are at least 6 inches inside the hood. Leave a workspace, which is not directly over the components, left open for the actual manipulations to take place. This will ensure that first air is never interrupted by an item placed in the DCA. Stage or place items on either side of this open area to avoid disruption of airflow.

Equipment Used in Aseptic Manipulations

Good hand placement is essential to proper aseptic technique. Not only must the technician ensure that the "first air" is not compromised, but there are critical areas of the equipment that must never be touched. For example, when working with a syringe, the plunger and tip should never be touched. Needle hubs should also never be touched. If these areas are touched or blocked from first air, they can become contaminated.

To properly attach a needle to a syringe, remove the protective outer wrapping without compromising the critical areas. When pulling back the plunger of the syringe, hold only the flat knob at the end.

Ampule necks and vial tops should be disinfected with sterile 70% IPA swabs. This should be done by making one gentle stroke across the surface, disposing of the swab, and allowing the area to dry. These surfaces are considered *critical sites* because they are a fluid pathway surface. They should be wet for at least 10 seconds and allowed to dry so that microorganisms are eliminated (discussed in Chapter 6). Equipment, such as needles, syringes, and tubing, is packaged in protective covering from the manufacturer and is disposable.

Many syringes are manufactured with a locking mechanism designed to connect to the needle. When you attach a needle to this Luer-Lok system, it requires a slight

TECH NOTE!
Remember to think of the DCA as clean air flowing toward the operator that has been filtered and should never be interrupted by hands or any object being used.

TECH NOTE!
Place all outer wrappings, paper, and excess garbage in the trash if possible or near the side of the hood. Do *not* place them in the DCA.

turn, and then the needle is "locked" into place. There are other syringes known as *slip-tip,* which just hold the needle on by friction.

REMOVING AN AIR BUBBLE

A common problem when using a syringe to withdraw a solution from a vial is that air bubbles can form in the barrel. These will prevent accurate measurements and must be removed.

First, hold the syringe upright and pull back the plunger slightly to allow a space for the bubble to go to the top. Firmly tap the sides of the syringe to allow the bubble to travel to the top. Expel the air in the syringe by slowly pushing the plunger up until the fluid fills the barrel completely. Read the measurement by looking at the rubber end of the plunger aligned with the graduations on the barrel.

A vial is a **closed system**, which means air is not free to go in and out of the container. Whenever a liquid is withdrawn from it, there must be an equal volume of air injected into it first. For example, if 3 mL of solution is needed, first inject 3 mL of air into the vial to replace this volume. This prevents a vacuum from forming and sucking the plunger back down, which will cause "spraying of the contents" upon withdrawal of the needle. If a **vented needle** is available, this procedure is not required because there will be no pressure build-up.

When inserting a needle into the rubber closure on a vial, the needle must never be "stabbed" into it. This can cause coring, which is when small pieces of the rubber closure get pushed into the solution and then possibly added to the bag. The needle should be placed at an angle with the bevel up. This will force the pieces away from the bevel. See Figure 7-1 for the step-by-step process to prepare a syringe.

Remember to ensure that first air is not interrupted, impeded, or diverted when setting up components in the DCA. Allow for approximately 6 inches between each item and 3 inches from the back of the hood. All supplies should be placed in the DCA so that clutter is reduced and maximum efficiency of workflow can occur. Now that we have discussed equipment, let's put this all together and prepare some admixtures.

Before performing any aseptic manipulations, always perform proper handwashing and garbing in the ante area, and once in the buffer area, clean the LAFW.

Setting up Equipment in a Laminar Airflow Workbench

ANTE AREA

- Perform all calculations or research required to prepare the medication ordered.
- Perform proper hand hygiene, garbing, and gowning procedure.

BUFFER AREA

- Spray hands with 70% IPA or disinfectant, allow to dry, and don sterile gloves.
- Spray gloved hands with alcohol, and allow to dry.
- Perform cleaning procedure for the LAFW.
- All supplies used in the DCA should be gathered and decontaminated by spraying or wiping the outer surface with sterile 70% IPA or removing the outer packaging at the edge of the DCA as it is entered into the aseptic workspace. This will aid in removing dust particles and any other contaminates.

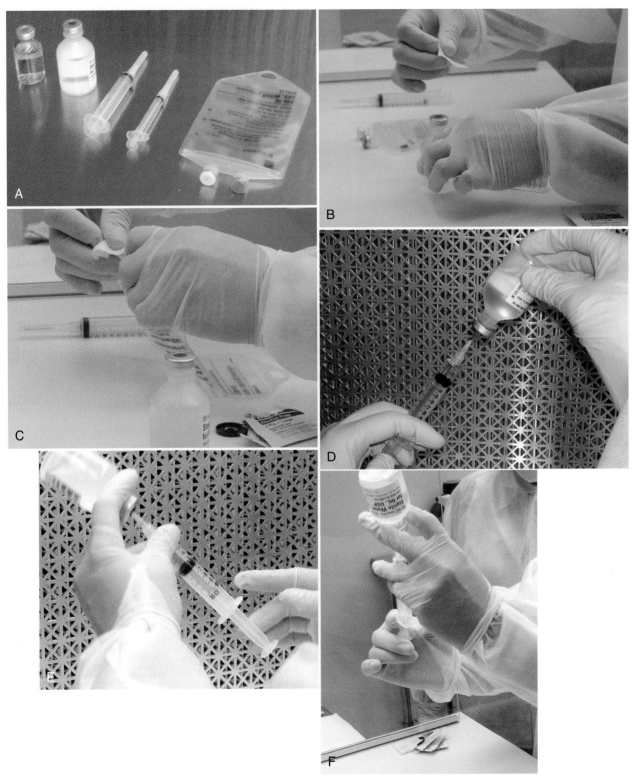

FIGURE 7-1 Steps showing how to prepare a syringe. **A)** Items placed in the LAFW hood, **B)** Clean vial top (critical area) with a sterile alcohol wipe, **C)** Clean the port on bag (critical area) with a sterile alcohol wipe, **D)** Add air to replace amount of fluid needed to withdraw, **E)** Withdraw fluid from the vial, **F)** Measure the amount needed in the syringe, **G)** Verify the amount in the syringe, and **H)** Add the drug to the port of the bag. (Courtesy of CriticalPoint, LLC, Gaithersburg, MD.)

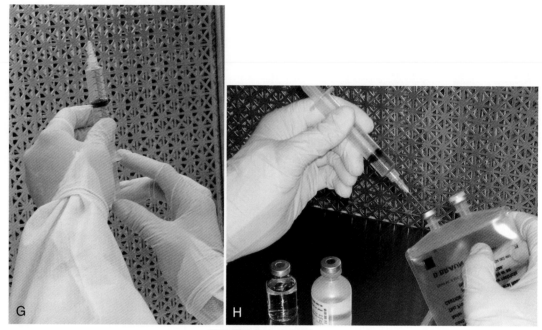

FIGURE 7-1, cont'd

- Attach the syringe to the needle inside the DCA without contact contamination or interruption of first air.
- Disinfect all critical sites using sterile 70% IPA alcohol wipes, and wait at least 10 seconds before use.
- Withdraw the correct volume of medication from the vial by injecting an equal or less amount of air into it first. (For example, if 2 mL are required, inject 2 mL of air into the vial and then withdraw the 2 mL of fluid.) Use the see-saw method to allow fluid and air to swap from the vial to the syringe.
- Replace the protective needle cover, and remove any air bubbles by gently tapping on the syringe. Air bubbles will cause the reading on the syringe to be inaccurate because it allows the air to take up space, and it reflects in the final measurement.
- Recheck all calculations.

If a medication is to be dispensed in a syringe, use the above steps to withdraw the contents and eliminate air bubbles. Attach a push-on or twist-on cap for delivery, and label.

Manipulations Used in Aseptic Preparation

"STAGING" OR PREPARING THE ADMIXTURE FOR THE PHARMACIST TO CHECK

To *"stage"* the admixture for the pharmacist to check, follow these steps:
- Remove the needle from the syringe, and place it in the sharps container.
- Lay the bag out with the stock bottle or vial of medication and the syringe drawn back to the amount of solution added to the bag.
- Initial the label, and check for a final time.

TRANSFERRING MEDICATION USING A VIAL WITH POWDER

Transferring medication using a vial with powder requires an additional step known as *reconstitution*. The powder must be mixed into a solution first in order to withdraw it from the vial.

Ante Area

- Perform all calculations or research required to prepare the medication ordered.
- Perform proper hand hygiene, garbing, and gowning procedure.

Buffer Area

- Spray hands with 70% alcohol or disinfectant, allow to dry, and don sterile gloves.
- Spray gloved hands with alcohol and allow to dry.
- Perform cleaning procedure for the LAFW.
- All supplies used in the DCA should be gathered and then decontaminated by spraying or wiping the outer surface with sterile 70% IPA or removing the outer packaging at the edge of the DCA as it is entered into the aseptic workspace. This will aid in removing dust particles and any other contaminates.
- Attach the syringe to the needle inside the DCA without contact contamination or interruption of first air.
- Disinfect all critical sites using sterile 70% IPA alcohol wipes, and wait at least 10 seconds before use.
- Add the correct fluid (diluent) to the vial according to manufacturers' recommendations. (If a vented needle is available, it is not necessary to add the equal volume of air.)
- Swirl or shake the vial to mix the powder.
- Once the powder is dissolved completely and using a needle and syringe, withdraw the required amount of solution from the vial, and remove any air bubbles as discussed earlier.
- Add the drug to the bag of fluid ordered and label.

TRANSFERRING MEDICATION FROM AN AMPULE USING A SYRINGE AND FILTER NEEDLE

Ante Area

- Perform all calculations or research required to prepare the medication ordered.
- Perform proper hand hygiene, garbing, and gloving procedure.

Buffer Area

- Perform cleaning procedure for the LAFW.
- All supplies used in the DCA should be gathered and then decontaminated by spraying or wiping the outer surface with sterile 70% IPA or removing the outer packaging at the edge of the DCA as it is entered into the aseptic workspace. This will aid in removing dust particles and any other contaminates.
- Attach a syringe to the filter needle or straw without contact contamination.
- Disinfect all critical sites using sterile 70% IPA alcohol wipes, and wait at least 10 seconds before use.

DID YOU KNOW?
Some medications, such as immune globulin, must not be shaken. Always refer to manufacturers' recommendations concerning preparation to find special mixing instructions about any medication.

TECH ALERT!
You must ensure that first air is not interrupted, impeded, or diverted when setting up equipment in the DCA. Allow for approximately 6 inches between each item and 3 inches from the back of the hood.

TECH NOTE!
Be careful at all times to not obstruct the first air with hand placement. Doing this will contaminate the surfaces of the critical sites and can cause infection for the patient.

TECH NOTE!
Remember to always be aware of possible incompatibilities between medications that can occur. These can be found in reference material, such as the *Handbook on Injectable Drugs*,[3] or on the package insert.

- Withdraw the correct volume of medication from the ampule by first holding the ampule upright and tapping the top to remove any solution from the head space.
- Swab the neck of the ampule with an alcohol swab, and grasp it with the thumb and index finger of each hand.
- Quickly snap the neck, being careful to direct the spray away from the HEPA filter.
- Remove the correct amount of solution from the ampule by tilting the ampule to at least a 20-degree angle. Position the needle in the shoulder area of the ampule, and pull the plunger back with the thumb and index finger of the opposite hand.
- Replace protective needle cover, and remove any air bubbles.
- Remove the filter straw or filter needle, and replace it with a standard needle before injecting the solution into a bag.
- Recheck all calculations.

ADDING MEDICATION TO A PLASTIC BAG

Once the medication is drawn up into a syringe and the bag port is swabbed with sterile 70% IPA, inject the medication into the bag and cover the port with a foil seal. Inspect the bag for particulate matter, such as coring, or any evidence of incompatibility. This may be a color change, cloudiness, haze, or solid particles.

Remove from the DCA, and label appropriately. Recheck all calculations. Once the admixture is ready, it should be labeled and "staged" with the needle removed, syringe drawn back to the added amount, and the stock vial that was used all placed together. Multiple-dose vials should be initialed, dated, and sealed with a foil seal. Discard any glass or sharp equipment in a disposable sharps container. Outer wrappings may be discarded in the regular trash.

ADDING MEDICATIONS TO A BOTTLE

Some medications are packaged in a glass bottle under a vacuum and sealed by a rubber stopper.

Ante Area

- Perform all calculations or research required to prepare the medication ordered.
- Perform proper hand hygiene, garbing, and gloving procedure.

Buffer Area

- Perform cleaning procedure for the LAFW.
- All supplies used in the DCA should be gathered and then decontaminated by spraying or wiping the outer surface with sterile 70% IPA or removing the outer packaging at the edge of the DCA as it is entered into the aseptic workspace. This will aid in removing dust particles and any other contaminates.
- Remove the foil seal from the bottle, wipe with a 70% alcohol swab, and allow to dry.
- Insert the medication into the bottle using a slight angle to prevent coring. The contents will be drawn in due to the vacuum effect.

Technicians preparing intravenous medications must use proper aseptic technique and environmental controls to ensure that products are safe for patients. Manipulations must be performed inside the DCA and airflow should not be disrupted. If a critical area is touched or first air is impeded, the technician must restart the process to ensure a safe and sterile product for the patient.

REVIEW QUESTIONS

1. What is the proper way to reconstitute a powder vial?
2. What is the proper way to transfer the contents of an ampule to a bag?
3. What is the proper technique for disinfecting the rubber closure on a vial or bag port?
4. Describe how to remove an air bubble from a syringe and correctly measure the solution needed.
5. Describe how to "stage" a completed admixture for the final check by the pharmacist.

CRITICAL THINKING

1. You have just prepared a stat order for a vancomycin IV. You have it "staged" and ready to be checked by the pharmacist when you overhear a nurse at the window requesting it. The tech from the front comes and asks when it will be ready? You reply, "I am waiting on the pharmacist to check it. So, it will be a few minutes." The tech insists that you made it correctly and that you should just let her have the bag. What would you say and why? Would a stat order override the need to make her wait for a pharmacist check? Explain your answer.
2. You have just prepared a large volume bag of normal saline (NS) with 4 mEq of sodium phosphate. The pharmacist on the floor has asked you to get it to him as quickly as possible. When you are staging the preparations for the pharmacist to check, you notice that one of the bottles is actually sodium acetate. Explain in detail what would you would do and why?

COMPETENCIES

TECHNIQUES FOR PREPARING
INTRAVENOUS ADMIXTURES

Evaluation Key: S= Satisfactory   NI= Needs Improvement

Name: _____   Quarter: _____   Date: _____

COMPETENCIES	STUDENT			INSTRUCTOR		
Student will be able to:	**S**	**NI**	**Comments**	**S**	**NI**	**Comments**
Discuss the use of a syringe and needle for aspect withdrawal of the contents from a rubber-capped vial.						
Discuss reconstitution of a vial with powder using the proper diluent.						
Discuss the use of filter needles and withdrawal of the contents of ampules.						
Identify all equipment and their proper use in various aseptic manipulations.						
Perform particulate matter inspection.						
Describe types of incompatibility to look for in a completed admixture.						
Identify appropriate times for checking admixtures to prevent medication misadventures.						
Describe how to "stage" (prepare for a final check) a completed admixture.						
Use reference materials to look for possible incompatibilities between medications.						
Interpret and perform calculations on an order for an intravenous medication.						
Discuss proper use of a sharps container.						

LAB ACTIVITIES

Name: _____   Quarter: _____   Date: _____

PROCEDURE: TRANSFERRING LIQUID CONTENTS OF A VIAL TO A BAG	EVALUATION		
	Student	**Preceptor**	**Comments**
Hood turned on at least 30 minutes prior to entering the ante area.			
Interprets order, and performs all calculations correctly in the ante area.			
Completes the garbing and handwashing procedures correctly.			
Uses lint-free wipes and 70% IPA, and performs LAFW cleaning.			
Disinfects all components/vials with sterile 70% IPA upon entering the DCA.			
Introduces only essential materials in the proper arrangement in the ISO Class 5 work area, or DCA.			
Does not interrupt flow of first air to critical sites (either by placement of materials or by placement of hands).			
Does not interrupt first air or allow touch contamination of critical sites.			
Performs all manipulations properly only in the appropriate DCA space.			
Adds appropriate amount of air to vial before withdrawing solution.			
Withdraws contents from vial without compromising first air or contaminating critical sites.			
Removes air bubbles correctly.			
Adds correct solution to bag appropriately.			
Affixes seal on bag port, and performs visual particulate inspection.			
Removes bag and all excess trash from the DCA, and disposes of sharps materials in appropriate container.			
Rechecks all calculations.			
Provides correctly-labeled admixture and appropriately stages equipment for final pharmacist check.			

Name: _____   Quarter: _____   Date: _____

PROCEDURE: RECONSTITUTING A POWDER IN A VIAL AND ADDING IT TO A BAG	EVALUATION		
	Student	Preceptor	Comments
Hood turned on at least 30 minutes prior to entering the ante area.			
Interprets order and performs all calculations correctly (including the diluent specifications).			
Completes the garbing and handwashing procedures correctly.			
Uses lint-free wipes and 70% IPA, and performs LAFW cleaning.			
Disinfects all components/vials with sterile 70% IPA.			
Introduces only essential materials in the proper arrangement in the ISO Class 5 work area.			
Does not interrupt flow of first air to critical sites (either by placement of materials or by placement of hands).			
Performs all manipulations properly only in appropriate DCA space.			
Adds proper amount of diluent to the vial per the manufacturer's recommendations.			
Allows contents to dissolve completely.			
Withdraws the correct amount of solution.			
Adds correct solution to the bag appropriately.			
Affixes the seal on the bag port, and performs particulate inspection.			
Removes bag and all trash from the DCA, and disposes of sharps materials in the appropriate container.			
Rechecks all calculations.			
Provides correctly-labeled admixture, and appropriately stages equipment for final pharmacist check.			

Name: _____   Quarter: _____   Date: _____

PROCEDURE: TRANSFERRING AN AMPULE TO A BAG	EVALUATION		
	Student	**Preceptor**	**Comments**
Hood turned on at least 30 minutes prior to entering the ante area.			
Interprets order, and performs all calculations correctly (including the diluent specifications).			
Completes the garbing and handwashing procedures correctly.			
Uses lint-free wipes and 70% IPA, and performs LAFW cleaning.			
Disinfects all components/vials with sterile 70% IPA.			
Introduces only essential materials in the proper arrangement in the ISO Class 5 work area.			
Does not interrupt flow of first air to critical sites (either by placement of materials or by placement of hands).			
Performs all manipulations properly only in the appropriate DCA space.			
Swabs the ampule and breaks it using the correct technique.			
Withdraws the correct amount of solution using a filter needle or straw.			
Attaches a regular needle to the syringe, and adds correct solution to bag appropriately.			
Affixes the seal on the bag port, and performs particulate inspection.			
Removes bag and all trash from the DCA, and disposes of sharps materials in the appropriate container.			
Rechecks all calculations.			
Provides correctly-labeled admixture, and appropriately stages equipment for final pharmacist check.			

Bibliography

1. Pharmaceutical compounding-sterile preparations (general information chapter 797). In: The United States Pharmacopeia, 27th rev. and The National Formulary, 22nd ed Rockville, MD: The United States Pharmacopeial Convention, 2004; 2350-70.
2. Gahart BL, Nazareno AR. *2007 Intravenous medications,* ed 23, St Louis, 2007, Mosby.
3. Phillips LD. *Manual of I.V. therapeutics,* ed 4, Philadelphia, 2005, F.A. Davis Company.
4. Trissel LA: *Handbook on injectable drugs,* ed 15, Bethesda, MD, 2008, American Society of Health-System Pharmacists.

8

Total Parenteral Nutrition

TERMS & DEFINITIONS

Additives Drugs commonly added to an intravenous solution

Anorexia Extreme loss of appetitive

Hypermetabolic states Condition in which an abnormal rate of metabolism occurs, such as in trauma, fever, or severe burns

Hypoglycemia Abnormally low level of glucose in the blood

Kilocalorie (kcal) A unit of measurement in nutrition

Macronutrients A source of carbohydrates, protein, and fat

Malnutrition Any disease-promoting condition that results from either inadequate or excessive exposure to nutrients

Micronutrients Additives in a total parenteral nutrition (TPN), such as vitamins, electrolytes, and trace elements

Pancreatitis Inflammation of the pancreas

Peritonitis Inflammation of the lining of the abdominal cavity

Specific gravity Weight of a substance measured in grams per milliliters as compared to an equal volume of water

Total parenteral nutrition (TPN) Nutritional support in an intravenous preparation for patients who cannot take in sufficient calories due to trauma or certain diseases

INTRODUCTION

In this chapter we will discuss **total parenteral nutrition (TPN)** as well as the various components, preparation techniques, and calculation and storage information. There are many employment opportunities for technicians in the area of nutritional support. It is essential to understand the proper techniques as well as the goals of TPN therapy in order to prevent patient harm and provide the proper amount of calories required for a specific patient.

Patient Considerations and Rationale for Using Parenteral Nutrition Solutions

Nutritional imbalance occurs in patients who are not able to take in adequate amounts of nutrients through the gastrointestinal (GI) tract due to diseases or conditions, surgery, or trauma. Nutritional requirements for a patient can vary but commonly range from 2500 to 3000 calories per day while on TPN therapy, which is supplied in 2 to 3 liters of fluid daily. TPN solutions are intravenous admixtures that can be individually designed to meet a patient's nutritional requirements based on their disease or condition. These must be prepared using the highest quality of aseptic technique to prevent the spread of any bacteria that may be passed to the already critically ill or susceptible patient. They also can be very complex and require many calculations and manipulations.

The basic goals of parenteral nutrition are as follows:
- Replace nutritional deficits.
- Promote wound healing.
- Increase weight or diminish the rate of weight loss.
- Prevent protein or caloric **malnutrition**.
- Sustain nutritional balance during periods when oral or enteral feedings are not possible or sufficient.

TPN should be administered to patients who are malnourished or have the potential of becoming malnourished. Often, a good candidate has multiple problems, and TPN often follows a surgery or procedure where food intake is inhibited. Conditions can include:
- Chronic weight loss, such as from **anorexia** or chronic vomiting and diarrhea
- Conditions requiring the bowels to rest, such as massive bowel surgery, **pancreatitis**, or **peritonitis**
- Multiple trauma, coma, or critical illness (known as **hypermetabolic states**)
- Severe burns

Hypermetabolic states, like some of those listed above, require additional energy for the body to heal. A balance of nitrogen in the blood is essential to keep a balance of protein. A negative nitrogen balance is an indicator that lean body mass is being broken down faster than it is being replaced. When this occurs in malnourished patients, the body converts the protein to glucose (sugar) for energy. Conditions such as, fever, surgery, starvation, burns, and critical illness can cause metabolism to increase in an effort to speed up the healing process.

TECH NOTE!
For each gram of nitrogen loss over the amount the body requires for intake, 6.25 g of protein or 25 g of muscle tissue is lost.

DID YOU KNOW?

1 g of carbohydrate = 4 kcals.
3000 mL of dextrose provides 1000 calories.
For TPN orders, the physician will order the proper amount of calories he wants the patient to have daily and each macronutrient provides a certain amount. The amount of total fluid is important as well, so the best combination of volume and calories provided is determined.

DID YOU KNOW?

1 g of fat (Liposyn) = 9 kcal.
500 mL of 20% Liposyn provides 1000 calories per day.

Solution Components and Special Considerations When Preparing Admixtures

COMPONENTS

The components of TPN consist of an energy source, such as carbohydrate, a protein, and a fat. These three components are known as the base, or **macronutrients.** Sterile water for injection is also used to adjust the volume of the final solution.

CARBOHYDRATES

The major function of carbohydrates is to provide energy. The most common intravenous source for carbohydrates is glucose. When glucose in the form of dextrose is provided in a parenteral solution, it is completely bioavailable for the body without any effects of malabsorption. The highest concentration that should be given through a peripheral vein is 10% dextrose in water (D10W), and it should not be given for more than 7 to 10 days. This is considered peripheral parenteral nutrition (PPN) and is only used for short-term therapy in those whose normal GI functions will resume in 3 to 4 weeks. For TPN, a 20% to 70% solution of dextrose may be used. These solutions are administered through the central vein that leads directly to the heart due to their hypertonic qualities.

This provides calories that are essential to the patient for long-term therapy. If 20% to 70% solution of dextrose is stopped abruptly, **hypoglycemia** may occur due to an imbalance of glucose and insulin in the body due to the high concentration utilized in the solution. For this reason, TPN is started gradually and tapered off. A 10% dextrose solution may be required in some patients to allow for the dextrose load to level out.

FATS OR LIPIDS

Intravenous fats are primarily made up of safflower or soybean oil, egg yolks, and some glycerol to provide tonicity. Fat emulsions are available in 1.1 kcal/mL, which is a 10% solution and a 2.0 kcal/mL in a 20% solution. These solutions are known as the trade name, Liposyn, and they are a milky, white solutions.

Fat is a primary source of energy and heat. It provides twice as much energy calories per gram as either carbohydrates or proteins. It is essential for all structural cell membrane integrity. A condition known as *essential fatty acid deficiency (EFAD)* can occur, which causes complications such as impaired wound healing and an increased susceptibility to infections.

It is very important to carefully, visually inspect the fat emulsions for separation of the emulsion, and to not use them if there is a visible yellowish streaking.

PROTEINS

Proteins are body-building nutrients that promote the replacement of cells as well as tissue growth and repair. Protein can be found in scar tissue, antibodies, and even clots. Amino acids are the basic units of proteins and are used in the TPN solution. Some typical manufacturers' names are Aminosyn, Travasol, FreAmine, and Clinimix. These come in 3% to 15% solutions, and they are available with or without electrolytes.

ELECTROLYTES

Long-term TPN requires basic electrolytes, such as potassium, sodium chloride, calcium, magnesium, and phosphorus. Approximately 30 to 40 mEq of potassium is needed for each 1000 calories provided parenterally.

It is necessary for the transport of glucose and amino acids across the cell membranes. It may be given in the following ways:

- Potassium phosphate
- Potassium acetate
- Potassium chloride

Other electrolyte amounts needed are:

- Calcium gluconate or chloride: 10 to 15 mEq in 24 hours
- Sodium chloride or acetate: 60 to 100 mEq in 24 hours (maintains acid-base balance)
- Magnesium sulfate: 10 to 20 mEq every 24 hours

These are compounded and calculated specifically for each TPN according to blood levels, acid-base balances, and disease states.

VITAMINS

Certain diseases or other conditions can alter the amount of vitamins available in the body, and this deficiency can cause death to a critically ill patient. Vitamins, such as K1 (phytonadione), are found in lipids and, therefore, do not require additional injections to the patient if the patient receives this in the total parenteral admixture.

TRACE ELEMENTS

These elements or microelements are found in the body in minute amounts and are beneficial in many ways. Each element is a single chemical and has its own deficiency state. Zinc aids in wound healing, copper reduces iron absorption, and iron is needed for hemoglobin production, the main component of red blood cells. Other elements such as selenium are important in the production of antioxidants, while fluorine and nickel are necessary for proper bone and teeth formation. Trace elements are available from the manufacturer in a single vial and are added to the TPN with the other macronutrients.

OTHER ADDITIVES

In addition to combining components of the base (carbohydrate, fat, and protein) and the ***micronutrients*** (electrolytes and vitamins) to form the TPN, other medications specific to each patient may be necessary. These may include insulin, heparin for blood thinning, and histamine-2 receptor blockers, such as famotidine (Pepcid), to prevent GI problems, such as stress ulcers.

Administration of Total Parenteral Nutrition

Once the order has been interpreted and the ingredients gathered, the TPN solution should be prepared using sterile aseptic technique in a certain order.

ANTE AREA

- Perform all calculations or research required to prepare the medication ordered.
- Perform proper hand hygiene, garbing, and gowning procedure.

BUFFER AREA

- Spray hands with 70% alcohol or disinfectant, allow to dry, and don sterile gloves.
- Spray gloved hands with alcohol, and allow to dry.
- Perform cleaning procedure for the LAFW.
- All supplies used in the DCA should be gathered and then decontaminated by spraying or wiping the outer surface with sterile 70% isopropyl alcohol (IPA) or removing the outer packaging at the edge of the DCA as it is entered into the aseptic workspace. This will aid in removing dust particles and any other contaminates.
- Attach syringe to the needle inside the DCA without contact contamination or interruption of first air.
- Disinfect all critical sites using sterile 70% IPA alcohol wipes, and wait at least 10 seconds before use.

First, the base is made. This consists of the macronutrients, which are the amino acids, the dextrose, and the fat or lipid for the three-in-one solution. Some TPNs will call for the lipid to be infused separately; in that case, just the amino acid and dextrose will be together in the bag. The order of mixing is very important because the dextrose and the fat should not be directly combined.

GRAVITY METHOD

Each component is spiked (there is a sharp point at the end of the tubing designed to puncture the rubber port of a bag or vial) and a special empty bag that holds either 2 or 3 liters is used. There are three leads attached to this bag that allow the fluid of each source to enter the empty bag by gravity. The empty bag will hold the components once they are added together, and then it will become the TPN. The fluids are transferred into the bag by hanging them up and allowing the calculated amounts to flow into the empty bag. Drawing a line with a Sharpie marker on the correct measurement before starting the flow indicates the amounts. The flow of each component is controlled by clamping off the lead of each piece of tubing.

AUTOMATED COMPOUNDER MACHINES

Automated compounder machines (also known as "compounders") can be used to make the base as well. These automated machines allow the fluids to be measured by specific gravity, and they are programmable. *Specific gravity,* or the weight of each substance measured in grams per milliliters as compared to an equal volume of water, is programmed in the machine along with the desired volume, and the exact amount for each solution is pumped into the empty bag. For example, the specific gravity of sterile water is 1.00 g/mL and dextrose is 1.24 g/mL because the sugar solution is heavier than water. There are many advantages to using the compounder machines; they are faster than the gravity method, there is less touch contamination, and they have better accuracy than the gravity method. Once the order is calculated, the pharmacist can input it into the system and generate a label automatically. Each bag is given a number, and the technician programs the compounder that sits directly inside the laminar airflow workbench (LAFW) and monitors the process. If there is a need to program the amounts of each source to be added, the technician can manually enter the volume to be added and the specific gravity of that source at the machine.

MICRONUTRIENTS

Once the base is prepared, it can be placed on the side of the direct compounding area (DCA), out of the way, and the other ingredients or micronutrients can be introduced into the DCA. Each one should be drawn up individually. The amount of micronutrients that can be added vary from one or two up to as many as fourteen. If the gravity method is used, these will be gathered and staged in the LAFW in proper order as described in the previous sections, "Ante Area" and "Buffer Area." Refer to the steps for drawing up a vial in Chapter 7 if needed.

TECH ALERT!
Automated compounder machines are kept in the LAFW, and all aseptic technique procedures are necessary during use. Follow manufacturers' guidelines when cleaning the equipment as well as while performing calibration to maintain the highest accuracy.

The technician should always refer to the printed information from the manufacturer regarding incompatibilities and order of mixing throughout this process. For example, potassium phosphate and calcium gluconate can precipitate if they are added too closely together. These individual vials should be drawn up and then verified by a pharmacist before adding them to the bag of base solution preparation, which was made earlier.

If there is an automated compounder machine available for adding the micronutrients, this procedure is slightly different; it can be programmed to add these components similar to the way the base is made.

Even though TPN is most often administered in a hospital setting, a patient may receive this therapy at home. For patients who require TPN due to postoperative or preoperative procedures that prolong nutritional needs, those patients who will not ingest adequate nutrients, or those patients who are unable to be fed by a feeding tube, a technician will prepare the TPN at a home infusion facility where they will be delivered, and a home health nurse will administer the solution using an infusion pump.

SPECIAL CONSIDERATIONS

The U.S. Food and Drug Administration (FDA) has special steps to decrease the risk of precipitation forming in a TPN solution. The storage is extremely important due to the increased risk of microbial growth due to the high dextrose content. Once prepared, the TPN should be refrigerated or used immediately. After they are hung, they should be infused or discarded within 24 hours. All parenteral nutrition should be filtered with a 0.2-micron filter. TPN solutions are administered through an infusion pump so that the rate can be controlled and gradually increased. Before infusion, TPN should be warmed to room temperature for approximately 1 hour. Patient care should include daily weight, vital signs, and various lab values every 4 to 6 hours. If TPN is stopped abruptly, a bag of D10W should be administered at the same rate that the TPN was being given until the patient's status can be evaluated. Labeling is necessary and includes all ingredients and amounts added to the bag along with the expiration, rate to be infused, and the proper signatures of the preparer and a pharmacist.

Due to the complexity of TPN orders, and the amounts of *additives* that must be combined, it is even more important to follow the strictest aseptic technique to avoid potential infections to critically ill patients (Figure 8-1). The more manipulations that need to be involved in the preparation, the higher the risk of contamination of the parenteral admixture. Technicians should be extremely cautious when calculating the amounts of the additives as well as observing proper technique and storage requirements.

HOME HEALTH

DATE

PATIENT

ADDRESS

TPN FORMULA:

AMImO ACIDS: ☐ 5.5% ☐ 8.5% ☑ 10%	mL	
☐ WITH STANDARD ELECTROLYTES	425	
DEXTROSE: ☐ 10% ☐ 20% ☐ 40% ☐ 50% ☑ 70%	mL	
(check one)	357	
LIPIDS: ☐ 10% ☑ 20%	mL	
FOR ALL-IN-ONE FORMULA	125	

FINAL VOLUME		mL
qsad STERILE WATER FOR INJECTION *400 mL*	1248	

Calcium Gluconate	0.465 mEq/mL	5	mEq
Magnesium Sulfate	4 mEq/mL	5	mEq
Potassium Acetate	2 mEq/mL		mEq
Potassium Chloride	2 mEq/mL		mEq
Potassium Phosphate	3 mM/mL	15	mM
Sodium Acetate	2 mEq/mL		mEq
Sodium Chloride	4 mEq/mL	35	mEq
Sodium Phosphate	3 mM/mL		mM
TRACE ELEMENTS CONCENTRATE	☐ 4 ☐ 5 ☐ 6		mL

Patient Additives:

☐ MVC 9 + 3 10 mL Daily

☐ HUMULIN-R *10* units DAILY

☐ FOLIC ACID _____ mg
_____ times weekly

☐ VITAMIN K _____ mg
_____ times weekly

☐ OTHER: *MVI 10 mL/daily*

☐ OTHER: _____

Directions:

INFUSE: ☐ DAILY

☐ _____ TIMES WEEKLY

OTHER DIRECTIONS:

_____

_____

_____

_____

Rate: ☐ CYCLIC INFUSION: " ☐ CONTINUOUS INFUSION: " ☑ STANDARD RATE:
OVER _____ HOURS " AT _____ mL PER HOUR " AT *104* mL PER HOUR
(TAPER UP AND DOWN) " " FOR *12* HOURS

LAB ORDERS:

☐ STANDARD LAB ORDERS
SMAC-20, CO2, Mg+2 TWICE WEEKLY
CBC WITH AUTO DIFF WEEKLY
UNTIL STABLE, THEN:
SMAC-20, CO2, Mg+2 WEEKLY
CBC WITH AUTO DIFF MONTHLY

☐ OTHER: _____
_____
_____

VALIDATION:

_____
DOCTOR'S SIGNATURE

Print Name: _____

Office Address: _____

_____

Phone: _____

WHITE: Home Health   CANARY: Physician

FIGURE 8-1 Sample total parenteral nutrition (TPN) order. (From Brown M, Mulholland JL: *Drug calculations: process and problems for clinical practice,* ed 8, St Louis, 2007, Mosby.)

TPN ORDER SHEET

HOME HEALTH   DATE

PATIENT   ADDRESS

TPN FORMULA:

AMINO ACIDS: ☑ 5.5% ☐ 8.5% ☐ 10%   400 mL
☐ WITH STANDARD ELECTROLYTES

DEXTROSE: ☑ 10% ☐ 20% ☐ 40% ☐ 50% ☐ 70%   350 mL
(check one)

LIPIDS: ☑ 10% ☐ 20%   200 mL
FOR ALL-IN-ONE FORMULA

FINAL VOLUME
qsad STERILE WATER FOR INJECTION 400 mL   1350 mL

Calcium Gluconate	0.465 mEq/mL	5	mEq
Magnesium Sulfate	4 mEq/mL	10	mEq
Potassium Acetate	2 mEq/mL		mEq
Potassium Chloride	2 mEq/mL	20	mEq
Potassium Phosphate	3 mM/mL		mM
Sodium Acetate	2 mEq/mL		mEq
Sodium Chloride	4 mEq/mL	30	mEq
Sodium Phosphate	3 mM/mL		mM
TRACE ELEMENTS CONCENTRATE	☐ 4 ☐ 5 ☐ 6		mL

Patient Additives:

☐ MVC 9 + 3 10 mL Daily

☐ HUMULIN-R _____ units DAILY

☐ FOLIC ACID _____ mg
_____ times weekly

☐ VITAMIN K _____ mg
_____ times weekly

☐ OTHER: _____

☐ OTHER: _____

Directions:

INFUSE: ☐ DAILY
☐ _____ TIMES WEEKLY

OTHER DIRECTIONS:
_____
_____
_____

Rate: ☐ CYCLIC INFUSION: "   ☐ CONTINUOUS INFUSION: "   ☑ STANDARD RATE:
OVER _____ HOURS "   AT _____ mL PER HOUR "   AT _____ mL PER HOUR
(TAPER UP AND DOWN) "   FOR 12 HOURS

LAB ORDERS:

☐ STANDARD LAB ORDERS
SMAC-20, CO2, Mg+2 TWICE WEEKLY
CBC WITH AUTO DIFF WEEKLY
UNTIL STABLE, THEN:
SMAC-20, CO2, Mg+2 WEEKLY
CBC WITH AUTO DIFF MONTHLY

☐ OTHER: _____
_____
_____

VALIDATION:

_____
DOCTOR'S SIGNATURE

Print Name: _____

Office Address: _____

_____

Phone: _____

WHITE: Home Health   CANARY: Physician

FIGURE 8-1, cont'd

LABORATORY AND OTHER ADDITIONAL TESTING REQUIREMENTS

The patient on TPN must be monitored closely by a pharmacist and nutritional specialists to ensure the amount of carbohydrates, protein, and vitamins and minerals, such as trace elements, are appropriate. Since the patient on TPN is dependent on it for their only source of nutrients, slight changes in the blood levels can indicate changes to the components are required. This has to be monitored through weekly and sometimes daily blood tests to check for levels in the blood. For instance, if the glucose level becomes too high because of too much dextrose in the TPN, this can cause the patient to be hypoglycemic, which can lead to death. The TPN order would need to be adjusted by a physician and a new bag prepared by the pharmacy according to the new order presented. If a particular micronutrient level such as potassium chloride is too high, the amount in the TPN can be decreased to the next bag. Pharmacy technicians must be aware of the constant monitoring and possible order changes with TPN in order to provide the patient with the proper nutrients at all times.

REVIEW QUESTIONS

1. How are TPN solutions usually administered and why?
2. Why is it so important to make the TPN solution in stages and be concerned with the order of mixing?
3. Would a patient who refuses to eat be a viable candidate for long-term TPN, and if so, why?
4. Why is periodic lab work important when administering TPN? Discuss the type of labs that are being done and why.
5. Discuss the three basic components of TPN and their purpose.

CRITICAL THINKING

HT: __152__ cm   WT: __62__ kg   Patient: _____

Adult *Total* Parenteral Nutrition Order Form (Central Line Only)

Date 3/3/13	Is central line access in place? [ ] No [√] Yes
Time 0630	Type __grosshong__ Date placed ____3/2/13

Please note: Prescribers must make selections in section 1-6 of form.

1. Base Formula (Check one)	2. Infusion Schedule
[√] Standard Base: dextrose 20% and amino acids (AA) 4.25% (D40W mL and AA 8.5% 500 mL)	Rate: __83__ mL/hour
[ ] Individual base: Dextrose_____% and AA____%:	**Cycling Schedule (home TPN only)**
(final concentration)	Cycle_____ mL fluid over _____ hours
OR	Begin at _____
Dextrose __% _____ mL	
AA ___% _____mL	

3. Standard Electrolytes/Additives	OR Specify Individualized Electrolytes/Additives	
Check here [√]	Specify amount of electrolyte	Check all the apply
NaCl 40 mEq / L	NaCl _____ mEq / L	[ ] Adult MVI 5 mL / day
NaAc 20 mEq / L	NaAc _____ mEq / L	[ ] MTE – 5 5 mL / day
KCl 20 mEq / L	NaPhos_____ mEq / L	[ ] Regular Human Insulin
Kphos 22 mEq / L	KCl _____ mEq / L	_____ units / Liter
CaGlu 4.7 mEq / L	KAc _____ mEq / L	[ ] Vitamin C 500 mg / day
MagSO4 8 mEq / L	Kphos _____ mEq / L	[ ] H-2 antagonist _____mg / day
Adult MVI 10 mL / day	CaGlu _____ mEq / L	drug _____
MTE-5 3 mL / day	Mag SO4 _____ mEq / L	[ ] Other additives
DO NOT USE IN RENAL DYSFUNCTION!	Maximum Phosphate (Na phos) _____	
	40 mEq / L or K phos 44 mEq / L _____	
	and maximum clearance 10 mEq / L	

4. Lipids (Check one)	5. Blood Glucose monitoring orders
Infuse lipids over 12 hours IV	Blood glucose monitoring every _8_ hours with
[√] 20% 250 mL every Tuesday/Thursday	sliding scale regular human insulin.
[ ] 20% 250 mL every day	Route (Circle one) **SQ IV**
[ ] 20% 250 mL every other day	**Sliding Scale** (Check one)
[ ] Other schedule	[ ] Sliding scale per T and T protocol
_____	[ ] Individualized sliding scale (write below)

Additional Orders (All patients)	6. Routine Laboratory Orders (Check all that apply)
1. Consult Nutrition Support Team.	[√] BMP, Mg, Phos every AM X 3 days then every Monday & Thursday
2. CMP, Mg, Phos, triglyceride, prealbumin in the AM.	[ ] Prealbumin every Monday
3. Weigh patient daily.	[ ] Metabolic study per RT (University only)
4. Strict I/O & document in chart.	[√] 24 hour UUN and creatinine clearance
5. Keep TPN line inviolate.	
6. If TPN interrupted for any reason, hang D10W @ current TPN rate.	

Physician Signature *Dr. Tom Pane*

COMPETENCIES

TOTAL PARENTERAL NUTRITION THERAPY

Evaluation Key: S= Satisfactory   NI= Needs Improvement

Name: Quarter: Date:

COMPETENCIES	STUDENT			INSTRUCTOR		
Student will be able to:	**S**	**NI**	**Comments**	**S**	**NI**	**Comments**
Discuss the five goals of TPN therapy.						
Discuss types of patients or conditions that would be appropriate for TPN therapy.						
Discuss the importance of nitrogen.						
Discuss three macronutrients and their importance.						
Discuss three micronutrients and their importance.						
Describe types of incompatibility to look for in a completed TPN admixture.						
Discuss storage and labeling of TPN.						
Use reference materials to look for possible incompatibilities.						
Interpret and perform calculations on an order for TPN.						
Discuss common problems associated with patient administration.						

LAB ACTIVITY

Name: Quarter: Date:

PROCEDURE: PREPARING TPN (GRAVITY METHOD)	EVALUATION		
	Student	Preceptor	comments
Hood turned on at least 30 minutes prior to entering the ante area.			
Interprets order and performs all calculations correctly.			
Completes the garbing and handwashing procedure correctly.			
Uses lint-free wipes and 70% isopropyl alcohol (IPA) alcohol, and performs LAFW cleaning.			
Disinfects all components/vials with sterile 70% IPA.			
Introduces only essential materials in the proper arrangement in the ISO Class 5 work area.			
Does not interrupt flow of first air to critical sites (either by placement of materials or placement of hands).			
Performs all manipulations properly only in appropriate DCA space.			
Prepares the base in the correct order and amounts to create a three-in-one solution.			
Receives a pharmacist check (for the base) before proceeding.			
Stages the micronutrients in the correct order without compromising first air in the LAFW.			
Withdraws the correct amount of each component, and receives a check from the pharmacist before proceeding.			
Adds all components to the TPN bag appropriately.			
Affixes the seal on the bag port, and performs particulate inspection.			
Removes bag and all trash from the DCA and disposes of sharps materials in appropriate container.			
Rechecks all calculations.			

Bibliography

1. Pharmaceutical compounding-sterile preparations (general information chapter 797). In: The United States Pharmacopeia, 27th rev. and The National Formulary, 22nd ed. Rockville, MD: The United States Pharmacopeial Convention, 2004:2350-70
2. Gahart BL, Nazareno AR. *2007 Intravenous medications,* ed 23, St Louis, 2007, Mosby.
3. Phillips LD. *Manual of I.V. therapeutics,* ed 4, Philadelphia, 2005, F.A. Davis Company.
4. *Taber's cyclopedic medical dictionary,* ed 22, Philadelphia, 2013, F.A. Davis Company.
5. Trissel LA. *Handbook on injectable drugs,* ed 15, Bethesda, MD, 2008, American Society of Health-System Pharmacists.

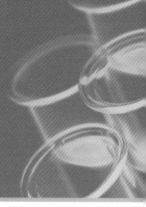

9

Chemotherapy Nutrition

1. Discuss cancer and common medications used in intravenous therapy, and discuss settings in which chemotherapy infusion would be appropriate.
2. Perform necessary techniques required to prepare chemotherapy solutions.
3. Describe special considerations, techniques, equipment, and precautions for working with chemotherapeutic agents.
4. Discuss education and training requirements for personnel handling hazardous drugs.

TERMS &
DEFINITIONS

Antineoplastic agent An agent that prevents the development or growth of malignant cells

Chemotherapy Treatment of disease with chemicals that destroy disease-causing cells

Chronic anemia Condition in which there is a prolonged loss of red blood cells

Cytotoxic agents Antineoplastic agents that kill dividing cells

Malignant Tending to or threatening to produce death; a neoplasm that is cancerous as opposed to benign

Metastasize Spreading of cancer cells to other organs or tissues

INTRODUCTION

The preparation of hazardous drugs requires special techniques, equipment, and training to ensure minimal exposure for the preparer and the patient receiving the medication. **Antineoplastic agents** or "cancer drugs" are designed to kill cancerous cells, but in the process, they also cause damage to healthy cells. All personnel who handle these medications must be aware of the risks and adhere to strict guidelines related to handling these products. With the ever growing population of the elderly, there are more patients requiring this therapy, and there is a growing demand for **chemotherapy** clinics that have technicians preparing these medications for hospitals, outpatient clinics, and home administration. In this chapter, we will discuss the most common types of medications being used in cancer therapy, proper techniques and equipment, and training guidelines to ensure technicians and patients will be protected.

Cancer and Cytotoxic Agents Used in Its Treatment

Cancer, or neoplastic diseases, involves abnormal tissues (neoplasm) that grow excessively through uncontrolled cell division (Figure 9-1). They can **metastasize** or invade the surrounding healthy tissues and cells interfering with their function. Antineoplastic drugs, also referred to as *chemotherapy agents,* are used to either destroy these cells or control their growth.

Chemotherapy drugs are designed to affect cells that divide and grow rapidly. Since the **malignant** cells have these fast-growing properties and a high metabolic rate, the chemotherapy drugs affect them more. However, cells of the oral mucosa, gastrointestinal tract, bone marrow, and lymph tissues also grow rapidly and are affected by these drugs as well. This is the main disadvantage of using these agents; they destroy normal cells as well as the cancer cells. If too much damage is done to the normal cells before the cancer is brought under control, sometimes withdrawal of treatment must occur.

There are also many side effects and complications associated with these drugs, such as severe pain, nausea and vomiting, hair loss, and a compromised immune system. Patients often have to receive additional supportive agents, such as epoetin alfa (Epogen, Procrit), to prevent **chronic anemia** that occurs due to the use of chemotherapy agents.

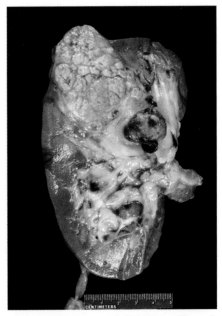

FIGURE 9-1 A cancerous tumor in an adult kidney. (From Leonard PC: *Building a medical vocabulary with Spanish translations,* ed 8, St Louis, 2012, Elsevier Saunders.)

These supportive agents are hormones that help to rebuild red blood cells that have been destroyed due to the medication. Since the chemotherapy medications are considered toxic or hazardous, special considerations must be observed when preparing them aseptically.

COMMON CHEMOTHERAPY MEDICATIONS USED IN CANCER TREATMENT

There are several classes of chemotherapeutic agents used in intravenous (IV) therapy. They are classified as the following:

- Alkylating
- Antitumor antibiotics
- Antimetabolites
- Hormones
- Enzyme inhibitors
- Immunomodulating agents
- Miscellaneous agents

Alkylating

These attach "alkyl groups," or side chains, to the proteins within the cancer cell and interfere with their function. Common drugs include:

- carboplatin
- cisplatin
- cyclophosphamide
- mechlorethamine oxide Mustargen, also known as nitrogen mustard N-oxide hydrochloride

DID YOU KNOW?
Nitrogen mustard was discovered as a result of experiments with poisonous gas during World War I.

Antitumor Antibiotics

These antibiotics interfere with the DNA or RNA synthesis. Common drugs include:

- bleomycin
- doxorubicin (Adriamycin)
- mitomycin
- dactinomycin (Cosmegen)

Antimetabolites

These substances replace, compete with, or antagonize a metabolic or body function by interfering with a specific phase of cell metabolism. Common drugs include:

- methotrexate (Rheumatrex Dose Pack, Trexall)
- fluorouracil (Adrucil)
- cytarabine
- gemcitabine (Gemzar)

Hormones

Hormones antagonize certain reproductive tumors and accessory tract organs by altering hormonal balance. Common drugs include:

- fulvestrant (Faslodex)
- leuprolide (Eligard, Lupron)
- triptorelin pamoate (Trelstar)

Enzyme Inhibitors

Enzyme inhibitors interfere with tumor enzymes. Common drugs include:
- asparaginase (Elspar)
- irinotecan (Camptosar)
- pegaspargase (Oncaspar)

Immunomodulating Agents

Immunomodulating agents inhibit growth of the cells. Common drugs include:
- aldesleukin (Proleukin)

Miscellaneous Agents

Miscellaneous agents are mitotic inhibitors, which means they interfere with cellular division.

Chemotherapy treatment can be administered in a hospital or inpatient setting as well as in an outpatient setting. It can also be accomplished by intermittent therapy where high doses are given weekly or monthly with a "rest period" in between. This allows the patient to gain strength and recover from some of the side effects that occur. Doses may be prepared in IV bags or as IV push in syringes. Common drugs include:

- ᵥᵢₙcᵣᵢₛₜᵢₙₑ (Vincasar)

gents

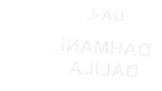

aring any IV admixture, but when : additional precautions. American and USP 797 have specific guide-)ecial procedures, disposal, storage, necessary exposure. Occupational roductive effects, and even cancer. :y cabinet (BSC) or compounding al hood takes air in at the top where irected downward toward the work :s not expose the operator to the air laminar airflow workbench (LAFW) outside air though HEPA filtration nould also be placed physically away :o remain running twenty-four hours

epartment for chemotherapy infusion :e masks, eye protectors, hair covers, sterile chemo-type gloves is required ials. A special sharps container marked WASTE" or "CHEMOTHERAPY ised as well. Red disposal bags or bio-)f the regular trash bags. Place all waste generated in the BSC in a small sealed plastic bag before removing it from the BSC. A special leak-proof absorbent pad should be placed on the work surface of the BSC to catch any small spills that may occur during manipulations. Only necessary items used in the preparation of the admixture should be placed in the BSC, because any items exposed to open vials or ampules must be disposed of in the hazardous waste bags.

Special Considerations, Techniques, Equipment, and Precautions

First air comes from above the work surface instead of coming across it, as it does in a LAFW. Placement of items should allow for the air above each item to be unobstructed during any manipulations. As trash is accumulated, discard it to the side of the work space (inside the BSC) in a puncture-proof container marked as *hazardous*. Any opened liquids should also be discarded in this container. Other materials used, such as wrappers and alcohol swabs that have had minimal exposure, can be placed in a sealed plastic bag and transferred to a container outside of the hood.

If possible, open packaging, such as syringes, tubing, and plastic bags, *before* opening the hazardous drug itself. This will allow much of the trash to be thrown away in the regular bag and avoid additional costs for special hazardous waste disposal.

To avoid unnecessary exposure for the nursing staff and the patient, tubing should be primed before adding the cytotoxic agent to the IV bag. This is accomplished by allowing "clean" fluid from the bag to run through the IV tubing and attaching a Luer-Lok fitting device at the end before adding the cytotoxic agent to the bag.

Since spray often occurs with withdrawal of the contents from a vial, a closed system vial-transfer device (CSTD) is recommended. These devices are needleless and contain a 0.2-micron hydrophobic filter that allows the air to escape through the closed system rather than in the air. The spike end is inserted into the vial, a syringe is attached on the device by Luer-Lok, and the contents are withdrawn. If a CSTD is not available, there are some special considerations to observe when using a syringe and needle in the preparation and delivery of chemotherapy medications.

- Use caution to avoid pressure build-up inside the vial that may result in spray or leakage.
- When adding diluent to a vial, inject slightly less air into the vial than required to maintain "negative" pressure.
- Keep the access pin or needle in the vial when measuring the dose.
- Use syringes that are large enough that the solution drawn up does not take up more than three-fourths of the space to avoid the plunger from coming out.
- Use a steady, slow motion while holding back on the plunger when removing the syringe from the vial to avoid leakage or spray.
- When removing air bubbles from a syringe, clear any solution from the hub of the needle by drawing additional air into the syringe. Any excess drug should be expelled into a closed container, known as an *empty evacuated container (EEC)* (Figure 9-2), rather than expelling it into the air.
- In the case of an IV push order, *never* transport drug-filled syringes with needles attached. Replace the needle with a push-on or twist-on cap, being careful to not contaminate the surface of the cap or the syringe tip.

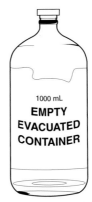

FIGURE 9-2 Empty Evacuated Container (EEC)

If an ampule is used, follow these guidelines:
- Tap down any drug from the top of the ampule, and put gauze around the neck when you break it.
- Change the standard needle to a filter device or filter needle prior to adding the solution to the IV solution container.
- Dispose of any remains of the ampule in the puncture-proof container that is marked *hazardous.*

Once the admixture is completed, the bag should be checked for leakage and wiped down with moist gauze. Wipe the entry port, and place it in a zipped-lock bag. It should be labeled with an additional warning label that reads *"Caution: Hazardous Drug. Handle with Gloves. Dispose of Properly."* on the drug container itself as well as the outside of the bag used for transport.

Hazardous drugs should be stored separately from other inventory to prevent contamination or unnecessary exposure and misadventures or errors, such as pulling the wrong drug. Wearing appropriate chemotherapy gloves is required when handling, stocking, distributing, preparing, and performing inventory control. Access should also be limited to only those personnel who are involved in hazardous drug preparation. When wearing double gloves, tuck the cuff of the inner glove under the gown sleeve, and tuck the cuff of the outer glove over the gown sleeve. If the outer gloves become contaminated, change them immediately. If the outer glove is punctured or torn, change both gloves.

CLEAN UP

Trained personnel must clean up spills immediately. Garb should include an outer pair of utility gloves and an inner pair of chemo gloves, gown, eye protection, and a respirator if aerosol droplets or powder is present. If a large spill occurs, the area should be restricted, and an absorbent pad should be used. There are standard chemotherapy spill kits available that include all of the necessary items needed to contain a spill, including protective gear and disposal bags. Spills on the skin should be washed with soap and water immediately, and contact with the eyes should be followed by a 3- to 5-minute rinse. All technicians involved in the preparation of hazardous drug products should be familiar with site-specific procedures and protocols.

TECH NOTE!
Never transport cytotoxic drugs through a pneumatic system.

TECH NOTE!
Follow these steps in this order for removal of gloves and gown once manipulations are complete:
1. Remove the outer pair of gloves in the BSC, and place them in a sealed bag.
2. Remove the gown.
3. Remove the inner pair of gloves, and discard all of the above in the hazardous waste container.

Education and Training Requirements

The ASHP and USP 797 have specific guidelines for handling hazardous drugs that include training and education guidelines. USP 797 states, "Personnel who compound hazardous drugs should be fully trained in the storage, handling, and disposal of these drugs" (USP). Training should occur prior to preparing or handling, and testing of specific techniques should be included at least annually. This should include didactic overview of drugs and ongoing training for new drugs, as well as safe manipulation practices, negative pressure techniques, correct used of CSTD devices, containment and clean up of spills, and exposure treatment.

Sampling of surface areas, such as the BSC and counter tops, at least every 6 months is also recommended for facilities that prepare large amounts of hazardous drugs. This is accomplished by using a swab to take a sample of the surface area to check for bacteria. Compounding personnel with reproductive capability should confirm in writing their understanding of the risks. The ASHP Technical Assistance Bulletin on Handling Cytotoxic and Hazardous Agents is also a comprehensive source of current information. It states, "Conduct regular training reviews with all potentially exposed workers in workplaces where hazardous drugs are used" (NIOSH). Disposal of all contaminated waste should follow federal and state regulations.

Always use proper aseptic technique when preparing any IV admixture. Extra precautions should be observed when handling hazardous drugs. All required personal protective equipment (PPE) (e.g., gowns, gloves, and masks) are always used and disposal of contaminated waste should follow procedures. Cleaning of the BSC should occur daily or when a spill occurs. All PPE should be worn to avoid contact with any hazardous drug residue. Patients with cancer have many additional complications and are very susceptible to infections due to compromised immune systems and general weakness. It is extremely important to remember to follow guidelines to safeguard yourself as well as your patient and other health care workers associated with hazardous drugs.

REVIEW QUESTIONS

1. Describe the procedure for using a CSTD.
2. When using a syringe and needle, discuss at least three special considerations that must be used to avoid leakage or spraying of aerosol droplets.
3. Discuss three guidelines from the ASHP and USP 797 for training requirements for personnel handling hazardous drugs.

CRITICAL THINKING

1. You are the chemo tech for the day at the hospital. It is time to put on your garb and prepare for the batch due this afternoon. When you start to put on your garb, you notice the gloves in the bin are not chemo gloves—but rather sterile gloves from the IV room. Can you double glove and use these instead? Explain your answer.

2. You must prepare a replacement chemo IV preparation for a patient whose line infiltrated and will need another one as quickly as possible. The nurse says she will wait, and you start. You are in a hurry and forget to take all of the necessary steps. You add air to the vial, which causes spray all over the bag as well as your gloves and sleeves. Explain what you would do in detail.

COMPETENCIES

CHEMOTHERAPY PREPARATION

Evaluation Key: S= Satisfactory NI= Needs Improvement

Name: Quarter: Date:

COMPETENCIES	STUDENT			INSTRUCTOR		
Student will be able to:	**S**	**NI**	**Comments**	**S**	**NI**	**Comments**
Discuss the main goals of chemotherapy.						
Discuss classes of IV antineoplastic agents used in treating cancer.						
Identify several examples of antineoplastic drugs.						
Discuss the BSC and how it works.						
List the PPE required when preparing hazardous drugs.						
Describe the procedure for priming tubing.						
Discuss inventory control, disposal, and storage for hazardous drugs and contaminated items.						
Describe the special techniques performed when using a syringe, a needle, and an ampule.						
Describe proper procedures for clean up and spills of hazardous drugs.						
Discuss the USP 797 guidelines for training and education.						

LAB ACTIVITY

Name: _____   Quarter: _____   Date: _____

PROCEDURE: PREPARING A CHEMOTHERAPY PREPARATION	EVALUATION		
	Student	**Preceptor**	**Comments**
Hood turned on continuously prior to use.			
Interprets order and performs all calculations correctly.			
Completes the garbing and handwashing procedure correctly (including double gloving).			
Uses lint-free wipes and 70% isopropyl alcohol, and performs BSC cleaning.			
Introduces only essential materials in the proper arrangement in the BSC work area (including absorbent mat).			
Does not interrupt flow of first air to critical sites (either by placement of materials or by placement of hands) or introduce aerosol or spray of chemo drug.			
Performs all manipulations properly only in BSC work space.			
Primes tubing with non-chemo solution prior to opening vial.			
Disinfects all components/vials with sterile 70% isopropyl alcohol.			
Prepares vial using a CSTD.			
Withdraws proper amount of solution.			
Adds drug, inspects for leaks, and wipes final admixture areas properly.			
Labels bag and outer bag properly to make them ready for delivery.			
Removes sharps and all trash from BSC (in a sealed, zipped plastic bag), and places materials in the appropriate container marked as "hazardous."			
Rechecks all calculations, and obtains final check from the pharmacist.			

Bibliography

1. Pharmaceutical compounding-sterile preparations (general information chapter 797). In: The United States Pharmacopeia, 27th rev. and The National Formulary, 22nd edition, Rockville, MD: The United States Pharmacopeial Convention, 2004:2350-70.
2. Gahart BL, Nazareno AR. *2007 Intravenous medications,* ed 23, St Louis, 2007, Mosby.
3. Phillips LD. *Manual of I.V. therapeutics,* ed 4, Philadelphia, 2005, F.A. Davis Company.
4. *Taber's cyclopedic medical dictionary,* ed 22, Philadelphia, 2013, F.A. Davis Company.
5. Department of Health and Human Services, Centers of Disease Control and Prevention, National Institute for Occupational Safety and Health: *NIOSH alert: preventing occupational exposures to antineoplastic and other hazardous drugs in health care settings* (website): www.microcln.com/PDF/2004_165.pdf. Accessed March 1, 2013.

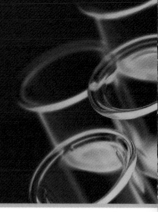

10

Patient Administration Considerations

INTRODUCTION

Pharmacy technicians work in a variety of settings, including home health and hospice care. Intravenous (IV) medications are most often prepared in a hospital setting, but they are also prepared in other facilities, such as home health agencies or doctor's offices, that have USP 797 cleanrooms where technicians prepare IVs for administration either as outpatient or home delivery. It is imperative to follow proper aseptic technique procedures to ensure the most sterile medication possible. In this chapter, we will discuss patient education and rights, common supplies used in home administration, and medication delivery devices or pumps that the technician will be responsible for.

Patient Education When Administering Intravenous Therapy in a Variety of Settings

Patients may receive IV therapy in a variety of settings, including home, hospital, long-term care facilities (e.g., retirement or nursing homes), doctor's offices, and even as an outpatient. No matter where the therapy takes place, there are always practices that health care workers, including technicians, should take to ensure patient safety and correct administration of medication. Patients should be informed about their therapy and equipment, and they should know what to look for to ensure that the medications are stable and stored properly. Technicians are a valuable part of this team and often are the personnel who maintain the equipment, gather the supplies needed, and prepare the medications for delivery.

HOME HEALTH CARE

Patient education is vital in the administration of IV therapy at home, and it should begin before a patient's discharge from the hospital. Patients should be instructed about the insertion of an IV catheter, peripherally inserted central catheter (PICC) line, or other implantable device that will be used to deliver the infusion. A PICC line can be used to deliver all types of therapy (Figure 10-1). These tiny tubes typically are used for 72 hours since they are inserted in veins close to the surface. Long-term therapy may require weeks, months, or even years, and special catheters designed to be inserted in the chest wall near the heart are used for this. These central venous catheters, such as Broviac and Hickman catheters, have been designed especially for longer duration therapy because they are inserted in larger veins very close to the heart and can stay in place for 1 to 2 weeks. If total parenteral nutrition (TPN) therapy is

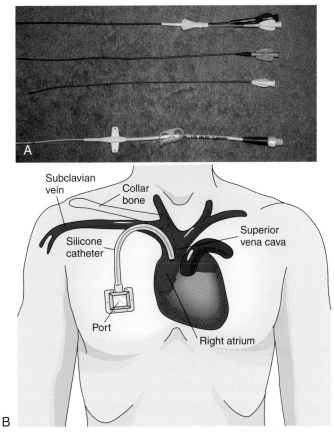

FIGURE 10-1 A, Peripherally inserted central catheter (PICC line). **B,** Central line with a Medi-Port. (From Perry AG, Potter PA: *Clinical nursing skills and techniques,* ed 6, St Louis, 2006, Mosby.)

required, an implantable infusion device, such as a Hickman or Broviac, may be needed. To insert one of these, the surgeon tunnels under the skin into the subclavian vein below the breastbone.

Patients with peripheral central catheters (PICCs) should be informed about signs of infiltration or phlebitis. This occurs when the solution leaks into the surrounding tissues and causes swelling, redness, and pain. Often the IV site must be rotated to prevent this from happening. Flushing the line should also be done by using the SASH method, which should also be explained to the patient. The SASH method helps the patient remember the steps that need to be followed to flush the IV line. The abbreviation stands for:

- **S:** 0.9% Saline flush
- **A:** Administer medication
- **S:** 0.9% Sodium chloride flush
- **H:** Heparin lock flush

Delivery of the supplies for home infusion will include enough heparin and saline to flush the line several times. Flushing the line is necessary after TPN, after intermittent medication infusion, after a blood infusion, and whenever a line needs to be locked. Patients and/or caregivers should also be informed about hygiene and handwashing, setting up the pump with medication, and troubleshooting problems, including 24-hour emergency numbers.

Delivery of all supplies should be timely and complete. Changes in temperature can affect the stability of the sterile preparations.

Refrigerated items should be shipped in coolers, and chemotherapy should be shipped in protective containers. The service should also include pickup of unused and waste items from the patient's home. Careful planning to include all supplies needed to administer the IV therapy will ensure timely administration without interruption.

TYPES OF INTRAVENOUS THERAPY

Chemotherapy infusion can be delivered through the intra-arterial route. The most common routes are the hepatic artery for colorectal cancer; the celiac artery for liver cancer; and the carotid artery for head, neck, and brain tumors. Compact, battery-operated, portable pumps are often used.

Pain management (such as morphine) can be given as a continuous or intermittent infusion. Intermittent dosing or patient-controlled analgesia (PCA) is common for hospice patients and is administered using a pump in which the patient can press a button to receive a dose of narcotics. The pump is preprogrammed in the pharmacy according to the physician's order and locked so it cannot be changed.

Antiinfectives can also be given at home and should include labs that monitor the patient's blood level to avoid toxicity. These should be given at specific intervals, are typically mixed as piggybacks, and can be given using computerized ambulatory pumps and syringe pumps.

Antifungals and **antivirals** may be administered at home using volumetric infusion pumps. These pumps deliver a measured amount and can be programmed accordingly.

TECH NOTE!
The technician who is preparing the medication for home delivery needs to know what type of IV line the patient has as well as how the medication is to be delivered, because the supplies to administer this treatment must be assembled and prepared for delivery along with the medication.

Investigational drugs are not approved for general use by the U.S. Food and Drug Administration (FDA). Guidelines, such as eligibility, monitoring for adverse effects, documentation, and disposal, are considerations for the use of these types of medications.

Infusion Pumps

VOLUMETRIC PUMPS

Volumetric pumps calculate the volume delivered by measuring the volume displaced in the reservoir (Figure 10-2). Special tubing is required and should be calibrated in milliliters per hour. Volumetric pumps are used for high-potency drugs because they are very accurate.

PERISTALTIC PUMPS

Peristaltic pumps move fluid by intermittently squeezing the IV tubing. These are primarily used for enteral feedings. They are calibrated in milliliters per hour.

SYRINGE PUMPS

Syringe pumps are piston-driven infusion pumps, which are critical for small doses of high potency drugs. The syringes are prepared in the pharmacy, and they can be administered in mg/kg per minute, mcg/min, and mL/hr. Syringe pumps are used most frequently for antibiotics and small volume parenteral drugs.

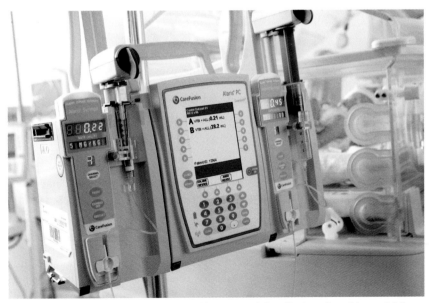

FIGURE 10-2 Volumetric pump. (Courtesy of CareFusion, San Diego, CA.)

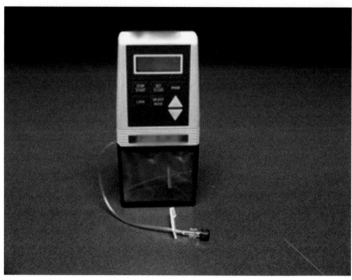

FIGURE 10-3 Patient-controlled analgesia (PCA) electronic infusion device. (Courtesy of CriticalPoint, LLC, Gaithersburg, MD.)

PATIENT-CONTROLLED ANALGESIA PUMPS

PCA pumps are used for pain management at home or in the hospital (Figure 10-3). They deliver medication through IV, subcutaneous, or epidural routes. The pump is programmed to deliver set amounts of the drug at certain intervals. A bolus dose, or demand dose, can also be programmed for breakthrough pain. This means that a set amount determined by the physician can be delivered by pushing a button when there is additional pain felt by the patient.

AMBULATORY PUMPS

Ambulatory pumps are lightweight and battery operated. They allow the patient to resume a normal life because they weigh less than 6 pounds. They can be used to deliver most infusion therapies. An example would include insulin pump therapy.

Technician Responsibilities in Infusion Therapy

According to the FDA Safe Medical Devices Act of 1990, all medical devices must be tracked, which includes infusion pumps. The pharmacy must know at all times the location of all their pumps by some means of a tracking system, such as logs, dates of service, or serial numbers. The Joint Commission requires that preventative maintenance is done once or twice yearly, or according to the manufacturer's recommendations and that cleaning is performed after each patient use. Technicians are generally responsible for these areas as well as the sterile preparation of the medications being sent.

TECH ALERT!
There is a special key, or a locking device, on PCA pumps to prevent a patient from receiving an overdose. There are specific settings, or modes, that must be programmed before the pump reaches the patient.

A typical log for checks on returned pumps might include the following:

ACTIVITY	COMMENTS	DATE
1. External inspection • Controls are in good working order. • Electrical plug/cord is good. • All doors work properly.		
2. Battery/power test • Plug pump in, and test it. • Test battery operation.		
3. Alarm check • Test pump to ensure that the alarm sounds when required indication occurs, such as pinched line or empty bag.		
4. Motor operations check • Insert an administration set. • Set volume to be delivered at 50 mL/hr. • Press run. • Check to ensure that the pump works properly to infuse the correct amount.		
5. Equipment cleaning • Clean with mild soap. • Disinfect with alcohol, and dry.		

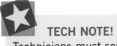

TECH NOTE!
Technicians must send the correct supplies and equipment to the patient's home to ensure accurate therapy. Remember, a patient's home has no nurses' station or cleanroom that the patient can go to for additional supplies like in a hospital setting.

All documentation should be accurate, timely, and always complete. Every entry should be signed and dated. In an office or home care environment, every conversation, follow-up visit, or set of instructions should be recorded. Nurses are using personal digital assistants (PDAs) for charting everything from labs, visits, patient care and progress notes, and discharge summaries in today's environment.

The technician who prepares the infusion for delivery is responsible for proper labeling and transport as well as gathering flushes and other supplies needed. The supplies needed depend on the infusion device being used, the route of administration (e.g., IV push or bag), the type of vascular device being used (e.g., a PICC line), and the type of drug therapy.

The pumps must be calibrated and maintained according to manufacturers' specifications. Delivery tickets should reflect an itemized list of all supplies delivered, because they are essential to accurate billing and quality patient care.

Examples of supplies sent to home for infusion therapy include the following:
• IV start kits
• Central venous catheter (CVC) kits, such as for PICC lines

- IV tubing
- Extension tubing (extension sets)
- IV filters
- Injection caps (these go on the end of the catheters)
- Syringes and needles (used to flush the line)
- IV pole (used for pumps that are non-ambulatory)
- Alcohol pads
- Infectious waste bags and sharps container for needles
- Tape (for dressing changes)
- Gloves
- Batteries
- Chemotherapy spill kit (if needed)
- Heparin vials (used to flush the line)
- Normal saline vials (used to flush the line)

In addition to preparing the sterile intravenous admixtures for home or long-term care use, a technician's role in home health care is slightly different from working in a hospital or retail setting. Other activities, such as gathering of all essential home infusion equipment and supplies (down to the last alcohol wipe), maintaining progress notes, or billing third-party administrators, are just as important. Cleaning, tracking, and maintaining infusion devices, performing quality control checks on various equipment, and even communication with family and other health care team members is essential for quality patient care. Since it is often family members or the patient who is administering the treatment, it is vital that all necessary supplies are provided and medication information is relayed to the patient to ensure the safest administration.

REVIEW
QUESTIONS

1. What kind of infusion is used to deliver cancer infusions, such as for brain tumors?
2. Which drugs are not approved by the FDA but can be infused at home?
3. Name two types of drugs that can be delivered at home using volumetric pumps for the prevention of infections following surgery.
4. What might hospice patients need to control pain at home?

CRITICAL
THINKING

1. If there were two patients named Mary Jones in your home infusion pharmacy, and the wrong Mrs. Jones received a delivery, how would you identify the correct one? What type of error would this be?
2. You have an order for morphine 1 mg/mL for a hospice patient. What type of infusion device would be appropriate, and why?
3. A home infusion patient calls to tell you that her metronidazole infusion that you delivered that morning is dark-colored and has crystals in it. Is this okay? If not, what could have happened to cause this?

4. A nurse at the home health agency notes in the chart, "The patient's right arm at the PICC line insertion is red and swollen." What does this indicate, and what action should be taken?
5. A patient is to receive TPN infusion therapy at home for 2 weeks. What type of catheter might be used, and why would it be appropriate?

COMPETENCIES

PATIENT ADMINISTRATION IN INFUSION THERAPY

Evaluation Key: S= Satisfactory   NI= Needs Improvement

Name: _____   Quarter: _____   Date: _____

COMPETENCIES	STUDENT			INSTRUCTOR		
Student will be able to:	**S**	**NI**	**Comments**	**S**	**NI**	**Comments**
Discuss types of infusion therapy.						
Identify several examples of infusion devices and how they work.						
Discuss infusion devices and what types of therapy they may be used for.						
Discuss the FDA Safe Medical Devices Act.						
Give examples of types of activities that would be found on a tracking record for a pump.						
Discuss types of supplies and equipment required for delivery for a typical home infusion therapy.						
Discuss the differences between a hospital IV technician's responsibilities and a home infusion technician's responsibilities.						

LAB ACTIVITY

Using the following home health order, create a supply list using the example given earlier in this chapter:

Vancomycin 500 mg/NS 250 mL q12h × 7 days

Note: Patient has a PICC line and will use a volumetric pump.

Bibliography

1. Pharmaceutical compounding-sterile preparations (general information chapter 797). In: The United States Pharmacopeia, 27th rev. and The National Formulary, 22nd ed, Rockville, MD: The United States Pharmacopeial Convention, 2004:2350-70.
2. Gahart BL, Nazareno AR. *2007 Intravenous medications,* ed 23, St Louis, 2007, Mosby.
3. Phillips LD. *Manual of I.V. therapeutics,* ed 4, Philadelphia, 2005, F.A. Davis Company.
4. *Taber's cyclopedic medical dictionary,* ed 22, Philadelphia, 2013, F.A. Davis Company.

11

Quality Assurance and Medication Error Prevention

1. Identify training and competency requirements for personnel who are compounding sterile preparations.
2. Discuss causes of medications errors and the technician's role in a prevention plan.
3. Define *quality assurance,* and list the major components of a quality assurance program.
4. Describe the compounded sterile preparation risk levels, including examples, quality assurance, and media fill test procedures.

Beyond use date (BUD) The date or time when a compounded sterile preparation (CSP) should no longer be stored or transported; it begins at the time of the preparation of the compound

International Organization for Standardization (ISO) Organization whose goal is to make products and services safe, reliable, and of good quality

Media fill test A test designed to access the quality of compounding processes or aseptic technique of personnel by using a microbiological growth medium

Process validation A systematic testing of aseptic technique and processes used in preparing CSPs to ensure sterility

Standard operating procedures (SOPs) Set of procedures, including environmental controls, personnel training, and validation of technique, to ensure sterility of all CSPs

INTRODUCTION

The roles of pharmacy technicians have changed greatly over the years. In addition to performing aseptic technique and routine prescription processing, the roles have expanded to more innovative responsibilities, such as administration in some states. Participating in medication error prevention and quality assurance (QA) programs have expanded the level of education and training as well as opened specialty areas. In this chapter, we will discuss the components of a QA plan and ways to prevent errors, the USP 797 guidelines for aseptic preparation, and the requirements for technicians and other personnel who prepare intravenous admixtures.

USP 797 Guidelines Concerning Risk Levels

Compounding sterile preparations requires proper techniques, equipment, and training. The Unites States Pharmacopoeia Chapter 797 (USP 797) as well as the American Society of Health-System Pharmacists (ASHP) technical assistance bulletin describes conditions and practices that will prevent harm, and even death, to a patient. Patient safety, accuracy, and the prevention of errors should be priorities in every aspect of the sterile preparation of compounded sterile preparations (CSPs). There should be *standard operating procedures (SOPs)* in place as well as a QA program to ensure that personnel involved in the preparation of CSPs are trained and that the environment and processes meet established criteria for accuracy. USP 797 states, "All personnel who prepare CSPs are responsible for understanding these fundamental practices and precautions, for developing and implementing appropriate procedures, and for continually evaluating these procedures and the quality of final CSPs to prevent harm." (USP)

Medication Errors

During preparation of CSPs, there are several types of errors that may occur. The most common error is microbacterial contamination, or nonsterility. This may be due to microbial, physical, or chemical contamination, such as improper handwashing, improper compounding environment, or incorrect manipulations or procedures. For instance, if handwashing is not done properly, contamination may occur due to physical contact.

If critical areas are compromised through either touch or interruption of first air in the laminar airflow workbench (LAFW), contamination may occur. If the LAFW is not cleaned properly or is not turned on for the required 30 minutes prior to manipulations, contamination may occur.

Any direct or physical contact with critical site areas poses the greatest threat of risk to the patient, and compounding personnel must always be conscientious of this fact. A technician *must* have a responsible attitude when performing aseptic compounding. Some errors may occur that would not be recognized by a pharmacist checking a final IV, such as the occurrence of a touch contamination (without being seen by the pharmacist), a wrong strength of an ingredient, or a syringe pulled back to the correct amount but not actually added to the admixture (Figure 11-1). Preparation usually occurs in the *International Organization for Standardization (ISO)* Class 5 area

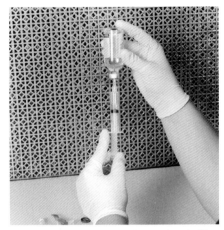

FIGURE 11-1 A syringe being held properly in the hood. (From Hopper T: *Mosby's pharmacy technician principles & practice,* ed 3, St Louis, 2012, Elsevier Saunders.)

TECH NOTE!

Remember: CSPs are potentially the most hazardous to patients because they bypass the digestive tract (oral route of administration) and are administered parenterally (into the bloodstream), which is one of the fastest routes of administration (Figure 11-2).

with minimal supervision of a pharmacist who is often staged in the order entry area or ante area. Final check of a retail prescription can easily include verification of the amount of tablets found in the bottle. How does a pharmacist measure the amount of additive in the admixture respectively?

Environmental conditions where compounding takes place must also meet certain standards to ensure sterility. Proper cleaning, placement, and environmental sampling should be incorporated to provide the cleanest environment for aseptic compounding. This is why the USP 797 provides environmental quality specifications and monitoring

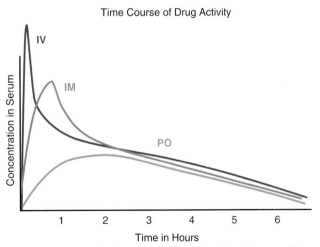

FIGURE 11-2 Routes of administration through the bloodstream. (From McKenry LM, Tessier E, Hogan MA: *Mosby's pharmacology in nursing,* ed 22, St Louis, 2005, Mosby.)

standards. Tasks, such as proper garbing and handwashing, air quality, and equipment calibrations, should be incorporated as standard procedures to prevent contamination and subsequent harm to the patient. USP 797 guidelines provide a sampling plan for air and surface compounding areas. These include areas within the ISO Class 5 area and surrounding surfaces, as well as the ISO Class 7 and 8 areas, which should be collected and reviewed on a periodic basis. Equipment should be kept in operating condition according to manufacturers' specifications. Accuracy of automated compounding devices, such as that used in total parenteral nutrition (TPN) preparation, and balances should also be tested to prevent errors in measurements.

Incorrect dosages and strength and quality of correct ingredients are also types of errors. Labels for CSPs should include correct amounts and names of all ingredients, total volume, appropriate route of administration, and storage conditions. Patient names should be double-checked, as well as all calculations, additives, and fluids used. All finished CSPs should be inspected for cloudiness or any particulate matter that may be present. Proper storage instructions and **beyond use dates (BUDs)** should also be included.

Medication errors can occur due to poor handwriting that is difficult to read, confusion about drugs with similar names, or a lack of training and knowledge of sterile technique and best practices. In the institutional setting, there are several ways to prevent medication errors. Some of them include:

TECH NOTE!
Use reference guides (e.g., Trissel's *Handbook on Injectable Drugs*,[5] *Drug Facts & Comparisons*,[3] and package inserts) for compatibility, dilution, and preparation and storage information.

- Recheck calculations and interpretations of orders. This may be accomplished by simply allowing another technician or pharmacist to read the same order.
- Reconfirm confusing or specialty orders. This may be done by reviewing websites (such as the Institute for Safe Medical Practices (ISMP) at http://ismp.org/) for high-risk drug information and sound-alike/look-alike drugs, or printed pharmacy references, such as *Drug Facts and Comparisons* or *Mosby's Drug Guide for Nursing Students.*
- *Always* check reference materials for unusual doses, and consult the pharmacist—especially for TPN or chemotherapy orders—before preparing the compounded product.
- Check for drug incompatibilities. Use reference sources, such as the *Handbook on Injectable Drugs* by Trissel or *2013 Intravenous Medications* by Gahart and Nazareno, to verify proper diluents, stability, and any special storage or preparation information.
- Do not store sound-alike drugs or look-alike drugs on the same shelf. Follow standards of practice and procedures to verify these drugs, and ask someone to check with you. For a complete listing of sound-alike/look-alike drugs, see the ISMP website (http://ismp.org/).
- Always work as a team to ensure the best patient care and continue to gain knowledge in the field. The IV technician is part of a team that should continuously look for ways to improve and expand knowledge about the quality of sterile preparations.
- Always continue to gain knowledge about new medications through continuing education and by staying current in the practice to ensure that the most up-to-date information and practices are used.

PATIENT RIGHTS OF ADMINISTRATION

Patient safety should always be the most important aspect of any health care worker's job, and patients are guaranteed certain rights when it comes to medication, including infusion therapy. They are as follows:

- *Right patient:* Be certain that names, birth dates, and any other identifying information specific to the patient is checked when interpreting the order and preparing the IV therapy.
- *Right medication:* Check the order for accuracy and completeness. Use references, such as Trissel's *Handbook on Injectable Drugs,*[5] and package inserts for dilution, storage, and mixing instructions.
- *Right strength:* Check the order for the correct dosage or strength, and label it accurately.
- *Right route:* Check references for the appropriate route, such as IV push, piggyback, or intramuscular (IM) injection.
- *Right time:* Verify the directions for the proper intervals for infusion, for labeling, and for the storage requirements.

Quality Assurance Practices and Quality Control Elements

A QA program consists of a way to monitor, evaluate, correct, and then improve all of the aspects of compounding sterile preparations. Anyone who is involved in the delivery of medication should be included in this QA process, including, but not limited to, technicians, pharmacists, physicians, nurses, and others in supportive roles. A QA program ensures that the quality of products and services meet a set of standards defined by the organization. This QA plan, or program, should include several components to ensure that the highest possible standards for compounding sterile preparations are met. The QA plan should include:

- A formalized plan in writing, which is provided to all of the appropriate personnel
- Adequate training, education, and instruction for all compounding personnel
- Performance competencies to validate techniques, such as routine evaluations of handwashing, proper garbing techniques, cleaning and disinfecting procedures, and aseptic manipulation skills (***process validation,*** a term used to describe the checking of the preparer's aseptic technique for sterility)
- Error prevention and medication awareness information
- A performance improvement plan to identify improvements or changes, solve them, and monitor their effectiveness
- Patient monitoring and reports of medication errors, adverse event reporting, and product defects

The QA program should evaluate the overall compliance regarding compounding sterile preparations SOPs, identify and analyze problems, and provide solutions or improvements to prevent medication errors or harm to a patient. Patients who receive home health infusion should also be provided with the contact information to report adverse events and product defects to the U.S. Food and Drug Administration (FDA) and the USP as well as to the compounding personnel. These reports should be reviewed periodically as part of the QA program in an effort to prevent future occurrences. If there are problems with manipulation or aseptic technique skills, printed materials (e.g., checklists or instructions provided during or after training) may be helpful. If deficiencies in procedures or technique are found, re-instruction and re-evaluation of the compounding personnel must occur. The quality of a product is determined at the time it is compounded by the person who is compounding it.[1] Proper technique, environmental controls and barriers, along with monitoring is essential to ensure that patients receive the proper medication.

COMPOUNDED STERILE PREPARATION RISK LEVELS

Compounded sterile products are categorized into three levels depending on their potential for microbial contamination or potential risk to the patient. Each level has its own conditions, such as environment, storage periods, QA procedures, and process validation requirements. Technicians must understand the risk levels as USP defines them in order to know what evaluation and procedures they require.

Low Risk Level Compounded Sterile Preparations

The low risk level CSPs are sterile products that are transferred to sterile containers, such as bags or syringes. The CSPs are compounded using sterile aseptic technique within an ISO Class 5 environment. Compounding consists of opening vials, transferring, measuring, and mixing of not more than three commercially-prepared, manufactured products. There may be no more than two entries into any single container or package. Examples include single volume transfers from a vial or ampule to a bag or bottle for a patient, or a single patient ophthalmic preparation. In the absence of a sterility test, the CSPs cannot be stored for more than 48 hours at controlled room temperature, or 14 days at cold temperature, or 45 days frozen. Sterility tests for low level CSP procedures should be included in the QA program for the facility. Other QA practices include routine disinfectant and air quality testing of the ISO Class 5 area, visual inspection of the CSPs upon completion to check for particulate matter and correct labeling, a review of all orders and ingredients, and an annual process validation for compounding personnel. This will consist of compounding a preparation using a ***media fill test*** for the drug, which is a growth-promoting soybean-based product. The soybean-based product is added to a solution in place of a drug, and then it is incubated for a period of time to allow for microbial growth if it is present.

In addition to a media fill test, personnel will be evaluated prior to compounding CSPs and before a media fill test by taking a sample of their glove fingertips and by observing their garbing, gloving, and handwashing procedures.

Medium Risk Level Compounded Sterile Preparations

The medium risk level compounds are prepared in low risk conditions (ISO Class 5), but they have one or more of the following additional conditions:
- Complex manipulations other than a single volume transfer
- Multiple small doses that are to be administered to multiple patients or a single patient multiple times
- Manipulations that take an unusually long time

TECH NOTE!

All of the procedures to prevent medication prevention errors do no good without a follow-up evaluation of why they happened and a solution to prevent them from occurring again.

Examples of medium risk level CSPs include preparing a TPN, transferring multiple ampules or vials of drugs into a single container, or filling the reservoir of injection and infusion devices, such as a morphine patient-controlled analgesia (PCA) cassette. In the absence of a sterility test, the CSPs cannot be stored for more than 30 hours at controlled room temperature, or 9 days at cold temperature, or 45 days frozen. Sterility test procedures should be included in the QA program for the facility. Additional QA practices for medium risk level CSPs include all of the low risk procedures along with a more challenging media fill test, which should be done annually.

High Risk Level Compounded Sterile Preparations

The high risk level is not seen in every facility and requires a much more in-depth media fill test. Nuclear pharmacies are an example of a type of facility for high risk level CSP products, such as radioactive products used in cancer treatment or medical procedures. Other types of high risk level compounding include using any non-sterile ingredients or containers, such as dissolving non-sterile bulk drug powders to make a solution, or measuring or mixing sterile ingredients in non-sterile containers before sterilization. An example would be preparing a CSP using bulk non-sterile morphine or another narcotic powder. In the absence of a sterility test, the CSPs cannot be stored for more than 24 hours at controlled room temperature, or 3 days at cold temperature, or 45 days frozen. In addition to all the QA practices for low level risk CSPs, a media fill test that represents high risk compounding must be done semi-annually.

Successful QA programs and medication error prevention is a team effort. Each and every person, especially those who are compounding, is responsible for ensuring the integrity of the final preparation. The process should include SOPs that outline tasks, environmental controls, validation methods, and provide education and training. Reporting of adverse events and a clear understanding of the aseptic technique for the medications used are essential to quality patient care. The five rights of the patient should always be a consideration when preparing any medication. Performance improvement programs allow health care team members to identify problems or errors, evaluate causes, develop solutions, and monitor the results. This, along with patient education, can greatly decrease medication errors.

As the roles of pharmacy technicians continue to expand, the specialty areas and administration opportunities will also increase. Technicians should always strive to gain knowledge in the field through participating in organizations, obtaining certification, and advancing education. The more knowledgeable the technician is, the better equipped he or she is at performing the correct practice. Continuing education for technicians is often free and can be found through a variety of sources. Organizations offering continuing education include:

- ASHP
- The Society for the Education of Pharmacy Technicians (SEPhT)
- American Association of Pharmacy Technicians (AAPT)
- National Pharmacy Technician Association (NPTA)
- POWER-PAK C.E.
- RxSchool
- Pharmacy Technician Certification Board (PTCB)

? DID YOU KNOW?
According to an article published by ASHP on CSPs, "The essence of quality assurance is proving that you are really doing what you say you are doing."[7]

TECH NOTE!
Technicians should be aware of their state's requirements for practice. For a complete listing of the state Boards of Pharmacy, go to the National Association of Boards of Pharmacy (NABP) at http://www.nabp.net.

Your facility is also a great resource for education as well as some state boards of pharmacy.

Patient safety is every health care worker's responsibility, and technicians should take an active role in QA programs and error prevention. This is the only way to ensure the safest and highest quality care for all patients.

REVIEW QUESTIONS

1. The most common error that may occur during the preparation of CSPs is contamination. Name three ways this may occur.
2. Discus the difference between an IV technician's responsibility level and how an error may occur and be missed when checked.
3. Medication errors can occur for several reasons. Name at least three different reasons and a preventative measure for each.
4. Define *QA,* and list six elements that should be included.
5. Name one type of CSP for each of the following:
   - Low risk level
   - Medium risk level
   - High risk level
6. Name at least three common practices associated with CSPs that should be evaluated on a periodic basis.
7. List the five rights of a patient.

CRITICAL THINKING

1. Discuss how you, as a technician, can participate in a QA program. Working at the technician level in a hospital system, name specific ways that you can improve patient safety, and give an example of a problem and a solution.
2. Explain the following statement in your own words, "All personnel who prepare CSPs are responsible for understanding these fundamental practices and precautions, developing and implementing appropriate procedures, and continually evaluating these procedures and the quality of final CSPs to prevent harm."

COMPETENCIES

QUALITY ASSURANCE AND
MEDICATION ERROR PREVENTION   *Evaluation Key: S= Satisfactory   NI= Needs Improvement*

Name: Quarter: Date:

COMPETENCIES	STUDENT			INSTRUCTOR		
Student will be able to:	**S**	**NI**	**Comments**	**S**	**NI**	**Comments**
Discuss the USP 797 guidelines regarding compounding personnel and their responsibilities.						
Discuss common types of errors that may occur when compounding CSPs.						
Identify several examples of errors that may not be noticed by pharmacist checking.						
Discuss USP's sampling plan for air and surfaces.						
List the items found on an IV label.						
List two references that may be used when compounding CSPs and the type of information found in them.						
List several ways to prevent medication errors.						
Given a scenario, describe a QA program and its elements.						
Describe a media fill test.						
Discuss low risk level CSPs, including some examples, storage, and QA procedures.						
Discuss medium risk level CSPs, including some examples, storage, and QA procedures.						
Discuss high risk level CSPs, including some examples, storage, and QA procedures.						

LAB ACTIVITY

You have been working as a technician student in a hospital pharmacy accredited by The Joint Commission (TJC) for about 2 weeks. One day while you are replenishing the operating room (OR) trays, you decide to look at a drug that you are not familiar with. When reviewing the package insert, you discover that the expiration date that is being marked on the labels on the vials in the tray is wrong. A homemade chart on the refrigerator that the technicians follow indicates the drug is good at room temperature for 30 days, but the insert says the drug is good at room temperature for *14 days.* Additionally, the drug becomes toxic after the 14-day time period, and more than 20 trays of this drug are currently on the OR floor.

Answer the following:

1. Why do you think this happened?
2. Could it have been avoided?
3. What were the correct steps that you, as the technician student, took?
4. Thinking about TJC guidelines and the components of a good QA plan, who should you tell first, and what should you do with the drugs in the trays on the OR floor?
5. What actions should follow this discovery to prevent it from happening again in the future?
6. Use the previous scenario to create your own QA program to prevent this from happening again. *Remember:* A good plan must have a way to monitor a process, evaluate what happened, correct it, and then improve the results or prevent the incident from happening again. Include all of the elements of a good QA plan including a summary of what happened, any patient consequences that could have occurred, a detailed description of the correct storage and expiration of this drug, and any processes that you would put in place, along with the required reporting elements for TJC. Your plan will be graded using the following chart:

Evaluation Key: S=Satisfactory   NI=Needs Improvement

Name: _____   Quarter: _____   Date: _____

COMPETENCIES	STUDENT			INSTRUCTOR		
Student will be able to:	**S**	**NI**	**Comments**	**S**	**NI**	**Comments**
Provide a specific, written, formalized QA plan, including the required elements to prevent this error from occurring again.						
In the QA plan, include training and education requirements for staff.						
In the QA plan, include specific drug information, including storage and expiration information.						
In the QA plan, include at least one new process that will ensure the identification of correct and current drug information for the department.						
Discuss the technician's role and training in the prevention of medication errors and participation in a QA program.						
Discuss reporting requirements for this scenario as it relates to The Joint Commission (TJC) and the pharmacy director.						

Bibliography

1. Pharmaceutical compounding-sterile preparations (general information chapter 797). In: The United States Pharmacopeia, 27th rev. and The National Formulary, 22nd ed, Rockville, MD: The United States Pharmacopeial Convention, 2004:2350-70.
2. McKeon MR, Peters GF. *VALITEQ aseptic technique validation system: compounding manual,* ed 2, Chicago, 2001, Lab Safety Corporation.
3. Bernstein WN. Codes + standards. Pharmacy facts. Architectural and environmental changes required for USP 797, *Health Facil Manage* 18(7):39-40, 2005.
4. *Drug Facts & Comparisons,* ed 67, 2012, Lippincott Williams & Wilkins.
5. Skidmore-Roth L. *Mosby's drug guide for nursing students,* ed 10, St Louis, 2013, Elsevier Mosby.
6. Trissel LA. *Handbook on injectable drugs,* ed 15, Bethesda, MD, 2008, American Society of Health-System Pharmacists.
7. Gahart BL, Nazareno AR. *2013 Intravenous medications,* ed 29, St Louis, 2013, Mosby.
8. http://www.ashp.org/s_ashp/docs/files/HACC_797guide.pdf

Glossary

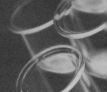

absorption: Movement of a drug into the circulatory system

additives: Drugs commonly added to an intravenous (IV) solution

admixture: The preparation of an IV medication that requires a mixture of medications

adverse effects: Drug effects that are unexpected and unwanted and are usually reported in only a few patients

anorexia: Extreme loss of appetitive

ante area: International Organization for Standardization (ISO) Class 8 area where personal hand hygiene, garbing, and staging of components, order entry, labeling, and high particulate activities are performed before entering the buffer area

antifungal: Medication that destroys or inhibits the growth of fungi

antineoplastic agent: An agent that prevents the development or growth of malignant cells

antiviral: Medication used to treat viral infections

asepsis: Condition free from germs, infection, or any form of life

beyond use date (BUD): The date or time when a compounded sterile preparation (CSP) should no longer be stored or transported; it begins at the time of the preparation of the compound

biological safety cabinet (BSC): Special hood where air flows downward through a high-efficiency particulate air (HEPA) filter; used for chemotherapy preparation

bolus: Also known as *direct injection* or *intravenous push (IV push; IVP);* small amount of medication injected into a port usually in an existing IV line (see also, IV push)

buffer area: International Organization for Standardization (ISO) Class 5 area where laminar airflow workbench (LAFW) or other primary engineering controls (PECs) are physically located and aseptic manipulations occur (see also, cleanroom)

Centers for Disease Control (CDC): United States Federal Agency under the Department of Health and Human Services concerned with control and prevention of diseases

chemotherapy: Treatment of disease with chemicals that destroy disease-causing cells

chronic anemia: Condition in which there is an extreme loss of red blood cells

clarity: Clear and free of visible particulate matter

cleanroom: Term sometimes used for *buffer area*

closed system: Used to describe a vial which is a sealed container of solution where air is not allowed to move freely in and out of the container

compatibility: Ability to combine drugs or substances without interfering with their action

compounded sterile preparation (CSP): Medications prepared using sterile technique

concentration: Amount of medication per amount of fluid

contamination: Introduction of pathogens or microbes into or on normally clean or sterile objects, surfaces, or spaces

coring: Breaking off small pieces of the rubber closure when withdrawing contents of a vial and allowing them to enter the solution or IV fluid

critical area: International Organization for Standardization (ISO) Class 5 environment where aseptic manipulations take place

critical site: Any location that includes fluid pathway surfaces, such as vial tops, bag ports, injection sites, or necks of ampules; areas to never touch, such as needle tips, tops of vials, and syringe plunger, to avoid cross-contamination during aseptic manipulations

cytotoxic agents: Antineoplastic agents that kill dividing cells

diluent: Solution used to dilute a powder form of an injectable medication

direct compounding area (DCA): Area within the International Organization for Standardization (ISO) Class 5 primary engineering control (PEC) where manipulations are performed (such as the laminar flow workbench [LAFW] and biological safety cabinet [BSC])

distribution: Movement of a drug through the body into tissues, membranes, and then organs

electrolytes: Dissolved mineral salts, usually found in IV fluids, such as total parenteral nutrition (TPN) or lactated Ringer's solution

epidural injection: Injection into the epidural space

excretion: Removal of a drug from the body

first air: Direct flow of air exiting the high-efficiency particulate air (HEPA) filter inside the direct compounding area (DCA), which should never be interrupted and is essentially particle-free

flow rate: Amount of medication to be infused over a specific period of time

garbing: Apparel or clothing that should be worn during aseptic preparation

gauge (ga): Size of the needle shaft (thickness); the finer the needle, the higher the gauge number

high-efficiency particulate air (HEPA) filter: Special filter used in the LAFW designed to remove 99.97% of particles that are 0.3 microns or larger. This creates a bacteria free environment to perform aseptic technique manipulations in.

hypermetabolic state: Condition in which an abnormal rate of metabolism occurs, such as in trauma, fever, or severe burns

hypertonic: Any solution containing a higher concentration of dissolved substances than red blood cells

hypoglycemia: Abnormally low level of glucose in the blood

hypotonic: Any solution containing a concentration of dissolved substances less than red blood cells

incompatibility: Drugs and drugs, or drugs and fluids, which cannot be put together due to the incident of unwanted or unexpected effects

International Organization for Standardization (ISO): organization whose goal is to make products and services safe, reliable, and of good quality

intra-arterial injection: Injection into an artery

intracardiac (IC) injection: Injection into the cardiac muscle or the heart

intradermal (ID) route: Injection into the dermal layer of the skin

intramuscular (IM) injection: Injection into the muscle

intrathecal (IT) route: Injection into the spinal canal

intravenous (IV) injection: Injection into the vein

isotonic: Any solution containing a concentration of dissolved substances, such as salts, that are the same as the concentration found in human red blood cells

IV push (IVP): Also known as *bolus;* small amount of medication injected into a port usually in an existing IV line (see also, bolus)

The Joint Commission: The shortened term for the Joint Commission on Accreditation of Healthcare Organizations; a non-profit, private organization that evaluates medical facilities to ensure good patient care

kilocalorie (kcal): A unit of measurement in nutrition describing a large calorie

lactated ringer's solution (LR): Sterile isotonic intravenous fluid used for electrolyte or fluid replacement

laminar airflow workbench (LAFW): Also known as the "hood." This area is designed to be used to perform aseptic technique in because it uses a HEPA filter to create an environment that produces sterile air

large volume parenteral (LVP): Containers of sterile solution used for intravenous medications; usually 500 mL to 3000 mL in volume

macronutrients: A source of carbohydrates, protein, and fat

malignant: Tending to or threatening to produce death; a neoplasm that is cancerous as opposed to benign

malnutrition: Any disease-promoting condition that results from either inadequate or excessive exposure to nutrients

media fill test: A test designed to access the quality of compounding processes or aseptic technique of personnel by using a microbiological growth medium

metabolism: Changing of the chemical structure of a drug by the body

metastasize: Spreading of cancer cells to other organs or tissues

micronutrients: Additives in a total parenteral nutrition (TPN), such as vitamins, electrolytes, and trace elements

microorganism: An organism, such as a bacterium, virus, or protozoan, of microscopic size

normal flora: Bacteria that resides on the skin's outer surface but does not cause disease

normal saline (NS): Sterile intravenous solution, also known as sodium chloride, used as a source of water or for fluid replacement

osmolarity: Number of dissolved particles in a solution per liter of solution

osmosis: Movement of a solvent (water) across a cell membrane from a lower osmolality to a higher osmolality

pancreatitis: Inflammation of the pancreas

parenteral: Any medication route other than the alimentary canal (digestive system)

peritonitis: Inflammation of the lining of the abdominal cavity

personal protective equipment (PPE): Equipment including shoe and hair covers, beard covers, gowns, masks, and gloves

pH: Degree of alkalinity or acidity of a solution. Acidity is usually between 0 to 6, whereas alkaline is between 8 to 14. Neutral pH is around 7.

piggyback (PB): Containers of sterile solution used to administer medications through a secondary set or intermittent infusion; usually 50 mL to 250 mL in volume

precipitation: Solid material or deposits that are separated from a solution often caused from reactions between drugs or drugs and certain fluids

primary engineering control (PEC): Controls such as laminar airflow workbenches (LAFWs), compounding aseptic isolators, or biological safety cabinets (BSCs) located in the buffer area

process validation: A systematic testing of aseptic technique and processes used in preparing compounded sterile preparations (CSPs) to ensure sterility

pyrogen: Fever producing substance

reconstitution: Used to describe the process of adding a sterile solution to a vial of powdered medication in order to make a liquid

secondary set: When a piggyback infusion is hung higher than the main IV solution which allows it to run into the vein faster. An example would be an antibiotic that would be ordered to infuse in 30 minutes.

side effects: Drug effects that are predictable, widely reported, and can be found in literature

small volume parenteral (SVP): Containers of sterile solutions used for intravenous medications; usually 50 mL to 100 mL or less in volume

specific gravity: Weight of a substance measured in grams per milliliters as compared to an equal volume of water

stage: Term used to describe how the final preparation is prepared for the pharmacist check of a sterile compound

standard operating procedures (SOPs): Set of procedures, including environmental controls, personnel training, and validation of technique, to ensure sterility of all compounded sterile preparations (CSPs)

Standard Precautions: Centers for Disease Control (CDC) guidelines that promote hand hygiene and the use of personal protective equipment (PPE)

sterile: Free of living organisms, especially microorganisms

subcutaneous route of administration (Sub-Q): Injection just below the skin into the subcutaneous fat layer

therapeutic effect: The intended effect of a drug

total parenteral nutrition (TPN): Nutritional support in an intravenous preparation for patients who cannot take in sufficient calories due to trauma or certain diseases.

United States Pharmacopoeia (USP): Non-governmental, not-for-profit public health organization that set standards for over-the-counter (OTC) and prescription medicines and other health care products in the United States; its main goal is to ensure public health

USP 797: Chapter in the United States Pharmacopoeia (USP) concerning parenteral medications compounding and equipment endorsed by The Joint Commission and American Society of Health-System Pharmacists (ASHP)

vented needle: A specialty needle used when compounding with vials of powdered medications that require reconstitution

A